Bariatric
Air Fryer Cookbook

A Methodical Guide For A Successful Long-Term Weight Loss After Bariatric Surgery. Discover 300 Air Fryer Low-Carb Recipes And Change Your Eating Habits Effortlessly

Amanda Kemp

© Copyright 2022 - All rights reserved.
Amanda Kemp

The content contained within this book may not be reproduced, duplicated or transmitted without direct written permission from the author or the publisher.
Under no circumstances will any blame or legal responsibility be held against the publisher, or author, for any damages, reparation, or monetary loss due to the information contained within this book. Either directly or indirectly.
Legal Notice:
This book is copyright protected. This book is only for personal use. You cannot amend, distribute, sell, use, quote or paraphrase any part, or the content within this book, without the consent of the author or publisher.
Disclaimer Notice:
Please note the information contained within this document is for educational and entertainment purposes only. All effort has been executed to present accurate, up to date, and reliable, complete information. No warranties of any kind are declared or implied. Readers acknowledge that the author is not engaging in the rendering of legal, financial, medical or professional advice. The content within this book has been derived from various sources. Please consult a licensed professional before attempting any techniques outlined in this book.
By reading this document, the reader agrees that under no circumstances is the author responsible for any losses, direct or indirect, which are incurred as a result of the use of information contained within this document, including, but not limited to, errors, omissions, or inaccuracies.

Table Of Contents

INTRODUCTION 8

CHAPTER 1: UNDERSTANDING THE BARIATRIC DIET 10
- Who Should Be On a Bariatric Diet? 10
- How Can I Lose More Weight After Bariatric Surgery? 10
- What Are Some Good Foods to Eat on a Bariatric Diet? 10
- What Are Some Good Drinks to Drink on a Bariatric Diet? 10
- What Foods Can I Eat When Taking Medicines to Manage Diabetes or Kidney Disease? 10
- What Foods Can I Eat to Manage High Blood Pressure? 10
- What Foods Should I Eat to Manage Kidney Disease? 11

CHAPTER 2: TIPS ON HOW TO START THE BARIATRIC DIET 12
- 1. Put a Plan Together 12
- 2. Set Up a Support System 12
- 3. Get Your Family on Board 12
- 4. Don't Get Discouraged if They Aren't Interested in Following the Plan With You 12
- 5. Know What You Want to Do 12
- 6. Make a Food Plan 12
- 7. Don't Beat Yourself Up if You Slip Up Once in a While on One of the Guidelines 12
- 8. Don't Be Afraid to Ask For Help 12
- 9. Don't Be Afraid to Change Anything That Is Not Working 13
- 10. And Finally, Know That the Bariatric Diet Should Be More Than Just Your Weight Loss Solution 13

CHAPTER 3: OVERVIEW OF THE 4 PHASES 14
- The Four Phases of Bariatric Surgery 14

CHAPTER 4: WHAT FOODS TO EAT AND NOT TO EAT AFTER BARIATRIC SURGERY 18

CHAPTER 5: HOW CAN THE AIR FRYER HELP IN THE BARIATRIC DIET? 20

CHAPTER 6: HELP IN CHOOSING THE BEST AIR FRYER ON THE MARKET 22
- Ninja Air Fryer Max XL 22
- GoWise 7-Quart Electric Air Fryer 22
- Dash Compact Air Fryer 22
- Philips Compact Air Fryer 23

CHAPTER 7: RECIPES FOR BREAKFAST 24
1. Strawberries Oatmeal 24
2. Tuna Sandwiches 24
3. Garlic Potatoes with Bacon 25
4. Chicken & Zucchini Omelet 25
5. Tomatoes and Swiss Chard Bake 25
6. Shrimp Frittata 26
7. Zucchini Fritters 26
8. Chicken Omelet 27
9. Scrambled Eggs 27
10. Almond Crust Chicken 27
11. Mushroom Cheese Salad 28
12. Shrimp Sandwiches 28
13. Mushrooms and Cheese Spread 28
14. Lemony Raspberries Bowls 29
15. Asparagus Salad 29
16. Zucchini Squash Mix 29
17. Bacon-Wrapped Filet Mignon 30
18. Pumpkin Pancakes 30
19. Onion Omelet 30
20. Sweetened Breakfast Oats 31
21. Veggie Quiche Muffins 31
22. Steel Cut Oat Blueberry Pancakes 31
23. Very Berry Muesli 32
24. Strawberry & Mushroom Breakfast Sandwich 32
25. Shakshuka Egg Bake 32
26. Ricotta Baked in the Oven 33
27. Poached Eggs Italian Style 33
28. Denver Egg Muffins with Ham Crust 33
29. Cheesy Slow Cooker Egg Casserole 34
30. Make-Ahead Breakfast Burritos 34
31. Magic Hot Cereal 34
32. Baked Broccoli and Eggs 35
33. Broccoli and Tofu Quiche 35
34. Cheese-Filled Acorn Squash 36
35. Cheesy Spinach Bake 36
36. Greek Yogurt, Granola, and Berry Parfait .. 36
37. Eggs Florentine 37
38. Mexican Scrambled Eggs 37
39. Spinach Omelet 37
40. Egg and Avocado Toast 38

CHAPTER 8: RECIPES FOR LUNCH 40
41. Easy Rosemary Lamb Chops 40
42. Greek Lamb Chops 40
43. Easy Beef Roast 41
44. Juicy Pork Chops 41
45. Tuna and Spring Onions Salad 41
46. Bacon-Wrapped Filet Mignon 42
47. Classic Beef Jerky 42
48. Flavorful Steak 43
49. BBQ Pork Chops 43
50. Crispy Meatballs 43
51. Juicy Steak Bites 44
52. Lemon Garlic Lamb Chops 44
53. BBQ Pork Ribs 44
54. Herb Butter Rib-Eye Steak 45
55. Honey Mustard Pork Tenderloin 45

56.	Simple Beef Sirloin Roast	45	115.	Bacon with Vegetables 67
57.	Seasoned Beef Roast	46	116.	Avocado with Eggs 67
58.	Beef Burgers	46	117.	Beef Steak Air Fryer 68
59.	Season and Salt-Cured Beef	47	118.	Chicken Breast Air Fryer 68
60.	Simple Beef Patties	47	119.	Delicious Chicken 68
61.	Baked Tilapia Cheese	47	120.	Simple Asparagus Treat 69
62.	Breaded Cod Sticks	48	121.	Eggs with Carrots and Peas 69

CHAPTER 10: VEGETARIAN RECIPES ... 70

63.	Shrimp, Zucchini and Cherry Tomato Sauce	48
64.	Honey Glazed Salmon	48
65.	Crumbled Fish	49
66.	Salted Marinated Salmon	49
67.	Sautéed Trout with Almonds	49
68.	Cod Fish Nuggets	49
69.	Creamy Salmon	50
70.	Baked Onion Cod	50
71.	Mussels with Pepper	50
72.	Cajun Salmon	51
73.	Breaded Flounder	51
74.	Caramelized Salmon Fillet	51
75.	Salmon Butter Crumbed	52
76.	Cajun Shrimp	52
77.	Vegetable Egg Halibut	52
78.	Deep Fried Prawns	53

CHAPTER 9: RECIPES FOR DINNER ... 54

79.	Brine-Soaked Turkey	54
80.	Oregano Chicken Breast	54
81.	Thyme Turkey Breast	55
82.	Chicken Drumsticks	55
83.	Lemon Chicken Breasts	56
84.	Parmesan Chicken Meatballs	56
85.	Easy Italian Meatballs	57
86.	Buttered Salmon	57
87.	Crispy Haddock	57
88.	Miso Glazed Salmon	58
89.	Ground Chicken Meatballs	58
90.	Lemony Salmon	59
91.	Crispy Tilapia	59
92.	Vinegar Halibut	60
93.	Crusted Chicken Drumsticks	60
94.	Spiced Tilapia	60
95.	Simple Haddock	61
96.	Breaded Cod	61
97.	Spicy Catfish	61
98.	Tuna Burgers	62
99.	Mushroom Pita Pizzas	62
100.	Turkey Meatballs	62
101.	English Muffin Tuna Sandwiches	63
102.	Pesto Gnocchi	63
103.	Crispy Prawns	63
104.	Sweet & Spicy Meatballs	63
105.	Vegetable Egg Rolls	64
106.	Steak with Cheese Butter	64
107.	Potatoes with Black Beans	65
108.	Lentils with Mushrooms	65
109.	Quick Eggplant Air Fryer Recipe	65
110.	Chicken and Avocado Recipes	65
111.	Grounded Chicken with Mushrooms	66
112.	Chicken with Avocado Mix	66
113.	Eggs with Vegs	66
114.	Chicken with Lettuce	67

122.	Delicious Air Fryer Cauliflower	70
123.	Spinach Quiche	70
124.	Yellow Squash Fritters	71
125.	Eggplant Parmigiana	71
126.	Air Fryer Brussels Sprouts	72
127.	Endives with Bacon Mix	72
128.	Creamy Potatoes	73
129.	Creamy Cabbage	73
130.	Asparagus & Parmesan	73
131.	Walnut & Cheese Filled Mushrooms	74
132.	Chard with Cheddar	74
133.	Herbed Tomatoes	75
134.	Spiced Almonds	75
135.	Leeks	75
136.	Asparagus	75
137.	Lemony Lentils with "Fried" Onions	75
138.	Cauliflower Steak	76
139.	Onion Green Beans	76
140.	Green Beans and Cherry Tomatoes	77
141.	Onion Soup	77
142.	Basil Parmesan Tomatoes	77
143.	Beef Chop Salad	77
144.	Roasted Veggies	78
145.	Cabbage Salad	78
146.	Potato Salad	78
147.	Spaghetti Squash Chow Mein	78
148.	Zucchini Lasagna Roll-Ups	79
149.	Roasted Vegetable Quinoa Salad with Chickpeas	79
150.	Mexican Stuffed Summer Squash	80
151.	Tomato Bruschetta	80
152.	Roasted Garlic Zucchini and Tomatoes	81
153.	Soba Noodle & Edamame Salad with Grilled Tofu	81
154.	Broccoli Casserole	81
155.	Chickpea and Feta Salad	82
156.	Eggplant Pesto Mini Pizza	82
157.	Lentil Vegetarian Loaf	82
158.	Spinach Lasagna	83
159.	Vegetarian Frittata	83
160.	Seitan Bites	83

CHAPTER 11: SEAFOOD RECIPES ... 86

161.	Grilled Sardines	86
162.	Crunchy Air Fryer Fish	86
163.	Tuna Zucchini Melts	87
164.	Buttery Cod	87
165.	Breaded Coconut Shrimp	87
166.	Codfish Nuggets	88
167.	Easy Crab Sticks	88

#	Recipe	Page
168.	Fried Catfish	89
169.	Zucchini with Tuna	89
170.	Deep-Fried Prawns	89
171.	Monkfish with Olives and Capers	90
172.	Salmon with Pistachio Bark	90
173.	Easy Prawn Salad	90
174.	Fried Fish Fingers	91
175.	Salmon with Mushrooms and Bell Pepper	91
176.	Cod and Chicken Broth	91
177.	Spinach with Tuna Fish	92
178.	Sweet Potato with Tilapia	92
179.	Kale with Tuna	92
180.	Spinach with Salmon and Seashells	92
181.	Paprika Mix Salmon	93
182.	Zucchini with Salmon Fillets	93
183.	Black Beans with Ham and Salmon	93
184.	Tuna Fish with White Beans	94
185.	Kale and Salmon Fillets	94
186.	Cod with Celery Stalk	94
187.	Squash with Salmon Fish	94

CHAPTER 12: SNACKS 96

#	Recipe	Page
188.	Tacos Crispy Avocado	96
189.	Apple Chips With Cinnamon and Yogurt Sauce	96
190.	Mozzarella Cheese Bites with Marinara Sauce	97
191.	Spanakopita Bites	97
192.	Vegan-Friendly Kale Chips	98
193.	Light Air-Fried Empanadas	99
194.	Whole-Wheat Air-Fried Pizzas	99
195.	Zucchini Chips	100
196.	Air-Fried Avocado Fries	100
197.	Chicken Nachos with Pepper	101
198.	Dark Chocolate and Cranberry Granola Bars	101
199.	Bacon Muffin Bites	102
200.	Brussels Sprout Chips	102
201.	Herbed Parmesan Crackers	103
202.	Cauliflower Crunch	103
203.	Lemon Pepper Broccoli Crunch	103
204.	Delicate Garlic Parmesan Pretzels	104
205.	Cucumber Chips	104
206.	Cajun Cauliflower Crunch	105
207.	Sprouts Wraps	105
208.	Pickled Bacon Bowls	105
209.	Curried Brussels Sprouts	105
210.	Crispy Cauliflower Bites	106
211.	Garlic Asparagus	106
212.	Crispy Kale Chips	106
213.	Crispy Squash	106
214.	Garlic Mozzarella Sticks	107
215.	Homemade Peanut Corn Nuts	107
216.	Divided Balsamic Mustard Greens	107
217.	Honey Roasted Carrots	107
218.	Roasted Bell Pepper	108
219.	Baked Potatoes with Bacon	108
220.	Chicken Thighs	108
221.	Corn-Crusted Chicken Tenders	108
222.	Simple Buttered Potatoes	109
223.	Roasted Coconut Carrots	109
224.	BBQ Chicken	109
225.	Pork Rinds	109
226.	Crispy Brussels Sprouts and Potatoes	110
227.	Duck Fat Roasted Red Potatoes	110

CHAPTER 13: DESSERT RECIPES 112

#	Recipe	Page
228.	Chocolate Mug Cake	112
229.	Chocolate Soufflé	112
230.	Chocolate Cake	113
231.	Choc Chip Air Fryer Cookies	113
232.	Doughnuts	113
233.	Cherry-Choco Bars	114
234.	Crusty Apple Hand Pies	114
235.	Nutella-Stuffed Pancakes	115
236.	Chocolate Donuts	115
237.	Blueberry Lemon Muffins	116
238.	Sweet Cream Cheese Wontons	116
239.	Saucy Fried Bananas	116
240.	Air-Fried Apple Pies	117
241.	Air Fryer Tostones	117
242.	Avocado-Chocolate Muffins	118
243.	Banana Bread	119
244.	Butter Cake	119
245.	Green Avocado Pudding	120
246.	Cheesecake with Ricotta	120
247.	Berry Crumble with Lemon	120
248.	Apple Treat with Raisins	121
249.	French Toast Bites	121
250.	Cinnamon Sugar Roasted Chickpeas	121
251.	Brownie Muffins	121
252.	Pear Sauce	122
253.	Sweet Peach Jam	122
254.	Warm Peach Compote	122
255.	Pan-Fried Bananas	122
256.	Blueberry Pudding	123
257.	Banana-Choco Brownies	123
258.	Dark Chocolate Oatmeal Cookies	123
259.	Pumpkin Pie Pudding	124
260.	Apple Dumplings	124
261.	Cinnamon Fried Bananas	124
262.	Peanut Butter Chocolate Chip Cookies	124
263.	Chocolate Keto Cheesecake	125
264.	Vanilla Ciabatta Bread Pudding	125
265.	Classic Baked Oatmeal	125

CHAPTER 14: LIQUID AND PUREED RECIPES ... 128

#	Recipe	Page
266.	Alcohol-Free Mint Mojito	128
267.	Sugar-Free Strawberry Limeade	128
268.	Hearty Mint Tea	129
269.	Orange and Apricot Juice	129
270.	Apple and Citrus Juice	129
271.	Blueberry Cacao Blast	130
272.	Cucumber and Avocado Dill Smoothie	130
273.	Spinach Green Smoothie	130
274.	Coco - Banana Milkshake	131
275.	Strawberry and Cherry Shake	131
276.	Chia Blueberry Banana Oatmeal Smoothie	131
277.	Banana-Cherry Smoothie	132
278.	Mango Smoothie	132
279.	Cashew Milk	132

280.	Pumpkin and Carrot Soup	133
281.	Banana Almond Smoothie	133
282.	Protein Spinach Shake	133
283.	Fresh Lemon Cream Shake	134
284.	Avocado Banana Smoothie	134
285.	Banana Cherry Smoothie	134
286.	Squash Soup	134
287.	Creamy Avocado Soup	135
288.	Celery Soup	135
289.	Cauliflower Soup	135
290.	Avocado Milk Whip	136
291.	Banana and Kale Smoothie	136
292.	Beef Purée	136
293.	Blueberry and Spinach Smoothie	137
294.	Broccoli Purée	137
295.	Easy Chocolate and Orange Pudding	138
296.	Herbed Chicken Purée	138
297.	Matcha Mango Smoothie	138
298.	Ricotta Peach Fluff	139
299.	Split Pea and Carrot Soup	139
300.	Herb And Melon Kefir Smoothie	139
301.	Kefir And Yogurt Banana Flaxseed Shake 139	
302.	Piña Colada Smoothie	140
303.	Green Mango Smoothie	140
304.	Peachy Greek Yogurt Panna Cotta	140
305.	Nutty Creamy Wheat Bowl	141

CHAPTER 15: 30 DAYS MEAL PLAN 142

CONCLUSION 144

Introduction

The bariatric diet is a specific type of weight loss, which stems from the ideas in the book "Eat and Run" by Scott Jurek. It is designed to help individuals who have obesity. In general, it helps them to lose weight, increase endurance for longer periods of time, decrease hunger, and control symptoms associated with metabolic syndrome. Before beginning a bariatric diet, you should discuss the specifics with your doctor first to make sure that it will work for you and that it will not cause your health problems to worsen. They are also certain types of foods that should be avoided while on a bariatric diet because they might lead to an increase in or worsening of health conditions such as diabetes or cardiovascular disease.

The bariatric diet should be followed for several months and should be adjusted according to your weight. It might sound difficult to follow every meal, but it is not. You just have to stay in control of what you eat and drink. That is why it is important that you start with a low-calorie intake such as 500 calories per day.

The large intake of protein in the bariatric diet provides satiety keeping you from eating more food and getting hungry again often. This results in a rapid drop in weight because one does not have much access to food. The diet also recommends that you eat a lot of fiber, which helps to keep the digestive system moving and prevents constipation.

The bariatric meal plan consists of foods high in protein, complex carbohydrates and fiber. A list of items that are allowed on a bariatric diet is as follows:

Milk, yogurt or cottage cheese with protein powder for breakfast. You can have an apple or yogurt with this breakfast but you can't have toast. Your mid-morning snack could be eggs or a hardboiled egg. You could have 3 whole eggs or just 1 yolk with 1 whole egg and 2 egg whites for your meal replacement lunch. You can have a banana, orange or tomato with this meal but you can't have potatoes for lunch. Your late-afternoon snack could be vegetables such as carrots and broccoli. For dinner, you can eat 1 cup of cooked beans, lentils, black beans or chickpeas with salad or a small portion of salad. You can have bread with chard, lettuce or cabbage but not potatoes.

Most people find that following the bariatric diet is not tough at all and even enjoyable. The benefits will last forever.

CHAPTER 1:

Understanding The Bariatric Diet

A bariatric diet is a diet created for someone who has had bariatric surgery. That person can also try the diet without surgery to lose weight. The diet uses foods and drinks that are lower in calories and carbohydrates. This type of food might help you lose weight by feeling full with less food, but it's not used to manage diabetes or any other health condition besides obesity.

Who Should Be On a Bariatric Diet?

Bariatric surgery is a common weight-loss option. Gastric bypass surgery is the most prevalent type of bariatric surgery. It changes the stomach and small intestine to limit the number of calories and nutrients your body absorbs from food. Another type of bariatric surgery you might know about is called sleeve gastrectomy. After this surgery, your stomach will be smaller but still can hold some food. If you have one kind of bariatric surgery or another, it's important to follow a diet created for that surgery—and to follow any other instructions from your healthcare provider after surgery, such as taking vitamins or supplements.

How Can I Lose More Weight After Bariatric Surgery?

You might be able to lower your calorie intake even more than you could after surgery. The size of your meal and portion size also might need to change. Ask your healthcare provider or registered dietitian (RD) for tips on healthy eating. In most cases, the weight-loss benefits of a bariatric diet will last for life, but you should keep losing weight until you reach a healthy weight for the size of your new body (based on the most recent definition).

What Are Some Good Foods to Eat on a Bariatric Diet?

You might be thinking that vegetables and fruits would be good choices. But these foods have more calories and carbohydrates than you need. Instead, use these foods as a side dish or in recipes: (1) lean meats and poultry, (2) fish, shellfish, and other seafood, (3) eggs, and (4) fruits.

What Are Some Good Drinks to Drink on a Bariatric Diet?

Water is the main beverage you should drink on a bariatric diet. The liquids will fill your stomach without adding extra calories or carbohydrates. If you need more liquid calories to stay full during meals, consider water with lemon squeezed into it or water with fruit juice added to it. Ask your healthcare provider if they're okay with this. If you want to switch from coffee or tea to water, do it slowly by adding more water and less coffee or tea.

What Foods Can I Eat When Taking Medicines to Manage Diabetes or Kidney Disease?

When you have these conditions, it's important not to suddenly change what you're eating. Instead, ask your healthcare provider about which foods the diet might include.

If you have diabetes and are on the meal plan for a bariatric surgery patient, make sure you know that the amount of food in each meal has been adjusted from the original plans. It will be lower than what you used to eat before taking your medicine. Ask your healthcare provider about this if you don't feel good after eating in a restaurant or dinner out.

What Foods Can I Eat to Manage High Blood Pressure?

High blood pressure, or hypertension, is a major cause of heart disease and stroke. Two types of high blood pressure are (1) primary care, in which your healthcare provider checks your blood pressure and tells you if it's normal or if you have high blood pressure, and (2) secondary care, in which you need treatment for high blood pressure.

In both cases, you need to follow strict guidelines for what you can eat. Ask your healthcare provider for more information.

What Foods Should I Eat to Manage Kidney Disease?
Kidney disease can lead to a number of health problems, including (1) high blood pressure (2) potassium levels in the blood and fluid in the tissues are both high, and (3) changes in your body's ability to process sugar. If you're having trouble with these symptoms, talk to your doctor about what you can eat. You might need to follow specific dietary salt, potassium, or sodium intake recommendations because these nutrients are important for helping your kidneys function normally.

CHAPTER 2:

Tips On How to Start the Bariatric Diet

A lot of people, especially those who have been toying with the idea, find starting a diet challenge. If you're having trouble eating, talk to your doctor about what you can eat. The Bariatric Diet is more than just about losing weight it's also about improving your general health and decreasing your risk of diabetes and heart disease. There are many steps involved in starting this type of diet which can get overwhelming for newbies trying to tackle it all at once. So, take things one step at a time and use these tips as tools as you go along.

1. Put a Plan Together
The first step to starting the bariatric diet is to make a plan for yourself. You will be building on these steps in the coming weeks, but this initial step is more about figuring out exactly what you want to achieve and why. Keep in mind that it may take several months or even years before you reach your goals. Make a plan now to reach those goals and give yourself realistic parameters within which you can work towards them effectively and comfortably.

2. Set Up a Support System
There are so many people who will be interested in seeing you following this diet, but it's great if you can find people who can help you make the transition. Whether it's your family or friends, finding a social group of people with similar goals is vital for making this change happen. In addition to supportive relationships, having a network of other weight loss experts to talk to and learn from is great.

3. Get Your Family on Board
Whether you are starting out on the diet with your spouse or even with your kids, getting everyone else on board will make sticking to the plan easier. You need your family's support in order to follow this diet and help ensure its success. This way you can also watch and learn from each other as you take individual steps towards better health.

4. Don't Get Discouraged if They Aren't Interested in Following the Plan With You
Changing one's lifestyle takes a lot of effort, so don't expect everyone else to be worried about doing the same. Don't expect them to follow the same plan you're following, especially if they don't want to.

5. Know What You Want to Do
Just because you make a plan doesn't mean you know exactly how to get there. If you have big career goals or decisions to make in your personal life, keep them in mind while doing the bariatric diet at the same time. This will help you make better choices about what is and is not significant. Eventually, when those other plans are reached, give yourself permission to take a break from whatever else is going on to focus on the diet for a while.

6. Make a Food Plan
Figuring out what you will eat and drink on this diet can be difficult. It is not as simple as deciding to stop eating at a certain time. You have to have meals, snacks, and drinks planned for the day, which can get complicated if you're trying to fit everyone in your family.

7. Don't Beat Yourself Up if You Slip Up Once in a While on One of the Guidelines
Don't get too upset over even small violations of portion control or hunger cravings that come with cutting down calories. Simply take what happened as a lesson and try your best to prevent it from happening again. (But if it does happen, get back on track as soon as you can.)

8. Don't Be Afraid to Ask For Help
There are so many health professionals available when you are on this diet, ranging from dieticians and nutritionists to personal trainers and gym owners. Don't feel the need to do everything by yourself. When you need assistance, ask for it and learn from what others have learned.

9. Don't Be Afraid to Change Anything That Is Not Working

You may find that one day you are eating relatively well, but then something different happens and your weight gain begins. What could it be? It could be as easy as a single meal containing all of your daily calories, or it could be that the snacks aren't what you're used to, despite consuming the necessary amounts of food at each meal.

If this happens and you're having trouble sticking to the diet, try changing things up a little to see if it helps. If nothing else works, go back to step number 1.

10. And Finally, Know That the Bariatric Diet Should Be More Than Just Your Weight Loss Solution

Remember that the diet is not just about losing weight. It's also about watching your blood pressure and cholesterol levels go down. It's about being able to see elimination foods in healthier quantities or not at all in your daily food choices. It's about increasing energy levels and developing better habits for a lifestyle that will last long after you've gone off this diet.

CHAPTER 3:

Overview Of The 4 Phases

Bariatric surgery is a weight-loss operation that reduces the amount of fat in a patient's body dramatically. It can help patients lose up to two or three times as much weight using less dangerous injections and staples than other weight loss treatments. The four phases of bariatric surgery are challenging and complex procedures that are different from one another in terms of complexity, length, nutrition options, risk factors, and outcomes. Bariatric surgeries can be lifesaving for many people suffering from obesity-related diseases such as diabetes or heart disease. There are several extra procedures that must be completed before laparoscopic gastric bypass and sleeve gastrectomy operations take place.

The Four Phases of Bariatric Surgery

Phase I. The Detoxification Phase

This is an overview of the patient and their history to determine whether or not they are healthy enough to be considered for surgery. In this stage, patients undergo lab tests, EKGs, and other tests as deemed necessary by their surgeon. The purpose of detoxification is to identify any possible health risks that could result in serious complications for the patient during or after surgery. During detoxification, patients also discuss issues with their surgeons about pre-operative nutrition and post-surgery diet planning with a dietitian. This gives them a realistic expectation of what their future eating habits will look like after surgery. It is also a time for patients to discuss how they plan on dealing with any mental health or dependency issues that they may have. The detoxification phase ends with pre-operative nutrition classes and diet consultation.

Phase II. The Pre-Operative Phase of Bariatric Surgery

This includes pre-operative testing, nutritional counseling and planning, and scheduling of the operation itself. Patients in the pre-operative phase speak with their dietitian about their eating plan following surgery as well as what dietary supplements they need to take to make sure that their body is healthy enough for surgery. The surgeon advises patients about what kind of physical activity is safe before surgery and which may be too strenuous. Phase II is also when patients take psychological tests to ensure that they are mentally stable before surgery. This requires a significant amount of follow-up and support from a psychiatrist. Some patients may receive counseling or psychotherapy during this phase as well. Phase II ends with patients completing an extensive physical examination with their surgeons.

Phase III. The Day of Surgery

Patients go into the hospital on the day of their operation and stay overnight. They are monitored to make sure they are doing well while passing through each phase of surgery. In this stage, patients have their bariatric surgery performed by surgeons under general anesthesia or deep sedation in most cases. Patients are monitored to make sure they are progressing satisfactorily through each step of surgery as well. Anxiety, depression, suicidal ideation, and cognitive difficulties are among the mental health issues addressed at this time. In the morning after surgery is completed, Phase III ends with patients going home where they recover for two weeks or longer depending on the nature of the case and their surgeon's recommendations. Some patients make it through Phase III in less than a week but most will be kept for a few days longer to ensure that their bodies recover from the surgery successfully.

Phase IV. Post-Operative Care

This phase lasts from one week or longer to several months depending on individual cases and surgeons' recommendations. In this stage, patients are put on a restricted diet that is designed to cause their bodies to adapt to the fact that they have lost weight. In some cases, this is done with the help of a low carbohydrate diet to limit the amount of glucose that enters the patient's body with every meal. Patients must continue to take prescribed medications, as well as dietary supplements, until instructed otherwise by their surgeons. This phase also involves counseling and physical therapy (PT) sessions with their surgeons throughout recovery. PT is performed in special recuperative beds so that patients can remain more comfortable while recovering in bed rather than on a regular bed. Phase IV ends when patients return home, which varies from one patient to another based on individual needs.

Pre-operative nutrition classes teach patients the basics of nutrition and what they should be eating before surgery. Patients are also counseled on how to deal with physiological changes that their bodies go through following surgery. They are advised that they will lose water weight as well as other liquids such as sweat and urine while they recover, which can cause some discomfort in the first couple of days or weeks. Some patients may experience issues such as acid reflux, constipation, and changes in their bowel habits after surgery.

Dietitians provide nutritional counseling during the pre-operative phase of bariatric surgery. Nutrition is an important aspect of the postoperative period, and patients will need to adjust their diet to match their bodies' caloric requirements. The pre-operative diet plan is designed with the help of their dietitian and nutritionist.

Before surgery, patients must make sure that they have prepared for the possibility that they may be restricted on what they can eat during and after surgery. Some patients opt for a liquid diet for this purpose, but others prefer the use of special forms of stool softeners such as liniments, suppositories or enemas if they have very little experience with eating proper foods in general or with regular diets such as liquid diets.

The pre-operative phase of bariatric surgery begins with patients scheduling the date of their procedure with their surgeons. Once the date is agreed on and accepted, patients must get approved by or have a financial guarantee approved by their insurance company. Most insurance companies require a consultation to confirm that they will cover the cost of the procedure before agreeing to it. Some may even require pre-operative testing such as psychological evaluations, blood tests, and certain other forms of testing before approving a patient for surgery. Some surgeons require that patients undergo these tests as well although other surgeons allow post-operative testing and only perform pre-operative tests when a patient's surgeon feels it is necessary. The pre-operative phase ends when patients get a chance to meet with their surgeons one last time before surgery. Some surgeons meet with their patients during the pre-operative phase but others do not.

The days before surgery include taking essential medications and dietary supplements to prepare the body for surgery. Patients are advised on what physical activity is safe for them as well as what activities may be too strenuous for them to perform safely once they have had bariatric surgery performed on them.

Pre-operative testing is performed by physicians in the pre-operative phase of bariatric surgery. Pre-operative testing is necessary to ensure that patients are in good health prior to the procedure. These tests are usually indicated by the patient's surgeon in order to make sure that they are healthy enough to undergo the surgery. Tests and treatments that may be performed include blood tests, an EKG, chest X-rays or CT scans, and psychological evaluations.

Post-operative physical therapy (PT) is usually done after bariatric surgery has been performed on patients. PT is used in addition to the other forms of treatment given at various stages of surgery such as antibiotics and calcium supplementation. The purpose of PT is to strengthen weak muscles that have been damaged by weight loss so patients can have a more active recovery period by working on their body's motor function without having to worry about becoming weak from not having worked out for too long.

If the patient's surgery results in an excessive amount of skin being removed at one or both ends of the abdomen, the surgeon may perform a skin graft from another part of the body. Patients are also given medications that contain propofol to prevent them from clenching their muscles for fear of causing pain or discomfort by doing so. Some patients are even given a local anesthetic that is injected into the hip or abdomen before bariatric surgery begins to reduce pain and discomfort during surgery.

Patients must be warned not to consume alcohol, especially wine and other alcoholic beverages because these substances tend to increase weight gain. It is also important not to consume food and drink that is too spicy since it can cause patients anxiety.

Patients are frequently startled to hear that following surgery their metabolic rates slow dramatically. This means that their bodies will digest food at a much slower pace, which can cause some discomfort at the beginning of recovery. In addition, patients are also prescribed laxatives during the pre-operative phase since excess weight slows down the digestive system of patients.

First Week. The first several days following bariatric surgery can be difficult for most patients and they must prepare themselves for this period by adhering to strict dietary guidelines. Patients must consume only liquids on the day of surgery and for the next five days afterward. Patients are allowed to slowly introduce food into their diet after the fifth day by starting with thicker liquids and then slowly moving on to regular foods.

During this time, patients are also exposed to post-operative exercise program so that they may better understand how their bodies will react to various workouts. This can help them know when it is time for them to stop exercising or change positions without feeling pain.

Second Week. Patients continue on with their post-operative routines as well as begin taking necessary medications designed for them by their physicians for them to gain a healthy amount of weight.

Third Week. Patients are still continuing with their post-operative routines as well as start working on strengthening their stomach muscles so they can finish eating the recommended amount of food. Patients are encouraged to have a healthy diet during this time in order to avoid any complications.

Fourth Week. By the fourth week, patients may start to attend pre-surgical get-togethers so they can come face-to-face with other patients who have had surgery performed on them. This helps build social skills while they are recovering and also helps them connect with others who are going through similar phases of recovery. Patients can also begin to participate in group exercise classes that they may have chosen to attend. These classes are designed so patients can gain a better understanding of their bodies and what they are supposed to be feeling during certain exercises as well as experience the benefits of weight loss.

Fifth Week. Patients may begin to work out more vigorously at this time as their body has aligned its needs with the requirements for physical therapy.

In most cases, bariatric surgery is considered a safe procedure. There are, however, some hazards linked with it. Bariatric surgery is done via laparoscopy or by open stomach surgery which is typically reserved for patients who have had previous abdominal operations performed on them within the past six months.

Patients are also required to follow dietary restrictions in order to achieve better results from the procedure. Dieting is required in most cases since weight loss is one of the primary goals of bariatric surgery. Most patients are encouraged to lose weight prior to their surgeries so they will be more comfortable throughout the surgical recovery period.

There are currently a lot of concerns about the safety of this procedure in regards to long term risks and effects. Some studies have shown that there is no difference in mortality between conventional surgery and bariatric surgery as far as heart disease, cancer, overall mortality, and other chronic medical problems go. However, other studies have shown that there is a higher incidence of cancer in patients who have undergone gastric bypass surgery.

Side effects are also common in cases where gastric banding is performed. These include the potential complications of vomiting, infection, bleeding, and postoperative bleeding. Vomiting may occur due to pain or discomfort after surgery. Patients may also experience nausea and diarrhea prior to eating as well as intense pain if they do not eat enough food.

It is also important for patients to be prepared for the possibility of post-operative complications when undergoing bariatric surgery. These complications can include electrolyte abnormalities which can cause dry mouth, trouble sleeping when properly aligned inside the body, and difficulty maintaining bladder control.

In cases where the procedure involves bypass surgery, patients should also be prepared for the possibility of blood clots and pulmonary embolism. Blood clots can occur during surgery if patients are not positioned properly during the operation. These clots may travel throughout a patient's body and cause damage to certain organs.

Patients should also be prepared for complication risks when they have undergone gastric banding. These complications can include infections, bleeding, varicose veins, skin breakdown, inguinal hernias, bowel obstruction, and even changes in their nutritional status due to malabsorption of food.

Patients who have undergone gastric bypass surgery are often required to take a number of medications in order to prevent complications. These medications include blood thinners, antibiotics, antifungals, pain medication and other dietary supplements.

There is also a small chance that surgery performed via a laparoscope may cause short-term complications such as pain, abdominal discomfort and nausea. This can be avoided if patients follow the instructions given by their surgeons during their surgical recovery. If there is some pain or discomfort occurring following the surgery, they should contact their physicians immediately. In addition, patients are advised not to drink any liquids after midnight 4 days before the surgery as well as eight hours prior to the operation.

Patients who were prescribed medications prior to surgery are also required to follow their doctors' prescriptions when taking them.

It is very important for patients to find an appropriate doctor and surgeon who can assist with their bariatric needs. Doctors should be trained in surgery as well as human anatomy and physiology. In addition, surgeons should also have a thorough understanding of the disease process being treated for them to perform the best possible surgery. Patients are also encouraged to request reports from their physicians describing the risks involved with each type of surgery.

You should contact a surgeon or physician right away if you have any other concerns or questions about the treatment. Many patients suffering from obesity and other related health conditions seek out bariatric surgeries to obtain the medical help they need. However, when they do, they will find that there are a lot of concerns involved with this type of treatment. Patients who wish to undergo the procedure should consult with their surgeons prior to the treatment.

CHAPTER 4:

What Foods to Eat and Not to Eat After Bariatric Surgery

If you are on any type of bariatric surgery, you will usually be on a meal plan to achieve your weight loss goals. While you can eat certain foods after surgery, others need to be avoided.

- **Foods to eat:** whole fruit, vegetables without skin or seeds, bananas, applesauce without sugar added, canned fruits in water or natural juices with no sugar added.
- **Foods to avoid:** fried foods, chocolate, coffee and tea (during the first few weeks), nuts, hard cheese, sour cream, mayonnaise (after six months), red meat.

Ask your doctor or registered dietitian what types of foods you can eat after surgery. They will tell you if you have had any type of gastric sleeve surgery or another type of bariatric surgery. There are some specific guidelines for each type of weight loss surgery.

While on your weight loss diet plan after bariatric surgery, be sure to drink plenty of water to avoid constipation. Every day, at least eight glasses of water should be drinking. You can also add lemon juice to your water for flavor. Stick to the meal plan and your doctor's recommendations.

There are certain foods that you should avoid after weight loss surgery. These include fried foods, nuts, chocolate and all fried foods. Your doctor will determine if you can eat any of these items after bariatric surgery.

You will need to start eating some new foods to help with your weight loss after surgery. Foods you should be eating more include vegetables, fruits and whole grains that are high in fiber. To increase your fiber intake with vegetables and fruits, be sure to drink plenty of water when eating those types of food products. Other vegetables and fruits that you can eat after surgery are broccoli, squash, cauliflower, Brussels sprouts, tomatoes and spinach.

Whole grain foods include oatmeal (brown), whole wheat bread and cereal. If a bread is made with whole grains, it will be clearly labeled as such on the packaging. Whole grain foods should be eaten without much fruit added or sugar such as jam or jelly. If a food product has sugar added to it (sugar-sweetened cereals) it should not be eaten after surgery because of its effect on blood sugar levels.

Vegetables and fruits may be eaten raw or cooked. Cooking vegetables and fruits can cause them to have different nutrients. If a vegetable or fruit has a core, it should not be eaten after surgery because fruits and vegetables with cores are more fragile. If a vegetable or fruit is leafy, it may be eaten after surgery if the skin is intact.

Whole grain breads often include up to three g of fiber per slice however, if the bread contains added sugar, that portion of the bread should not be consumed after surgery due to its influence on blood sugar levels. Some types of fiber supplements can also add extra fiber to your daily diet plan after bariatric surgery.

After surgery, you will usually eat smaller portions of food than you did before surgery. It is important to eat moderate portions of food in order to stay healthy. Sometimes the portion size is determined by your doctor, but most providers prefer you to make your portion sizes the same size as they were when you were overweight.

After bariatric surgery, some people are concerned that they cannot eat much at all after surgery. However, this is not true because everyone's calorie needs vary an obese person may need a few hundred fewer calories per day than a person who had never been overweight before.

After surgery, you will be consuming fewer calories than you did before. You must, however, ensure that you consume enough calories to meet your energy requirements. This is accomplished by eating foods that are high in fiber and protein. You should also keep your weight within a certain range so that your health will not be affected by weight loss surgery.

It is natural for many people to regain their weight after losing it through bariatric surgery. One of two things can cause this: 1) If a person does not adhere to the meal plan or 2) if the person's body senses that it is time for more nutrients such as protein. After surgery, people also experience cravings for foods that they were not able to eat before surgery, such as fried chicken, hamburgers and French fries.

It is important that you monitor your weight after bariatric surgery. Even if you've dropped a particular amount of weight, you should see your doctor on a monthly basis to see if the desired outcomes have been reached. The goal can often be different among individuals undergoing bariatric surgery because everyone's body responds differently to food manipulation (weight loss) and prevention of disease or illness.

Ask your doctor what type of surgery you had and the effects that different foods have on your body after surgery. Also, ask your doctor how much weight you should lose after bariatric surgery. Your doctors can tell you how many calories are in each food product that you eat after bariatric surgery and how many calories your body needs a day to maintain weight loss or maintain its current weight. If you've gained too much weight, it's time to alter your diet or seek fresh medical counsel.

CHAPTER 5:

How Can the Air Fryer Help in The Bariatric Diet?

Air Fryers are a relatively new little kitchen appliance that can change your life forever. The Air Fryer is relatively inexpensive, simple to use, and powerful enough to produce your favorite fried dishes guilt-free. Here are 9 ways that an Air Fryer can help you in your bariatric weight loss journey!

1) Air frying replaces deep frying - one of the most caloric cooking methods. Not only does it save you tons of fat calories, but it reduces cooking time by 25% or more! So now you have an excuse not to deep fry next time.
2) Reduced fat intake - the only way to have fried food without guilt, is instead of deep frying, you can air fry. And with just a fraction of the calories consumed in deep frying, it's easy to eat less fat.
3) Healthy fats: Air Fryer usage allows users to get more omega 3 fatty acids and other beneficial fats into their diet. What a great way to go!
4) Fiber, fiber, fiber - all that fried food can make you feel hungry sooner. Not so with air frying! You're not eating as much because these caloric fried meals are not that filling. Fiber is a weight loss key, and air frying helps in the fiber department.
5) Healthier fried food - if you have been eating fried food for many years, you can easily get away from it. No more struggles! Air frying will help in your bariatric diet goals every single time.
6) It's fun! - And not just because it's new, but it really is fun to make your favorite foods with less guilt and fewer calories. Once you start using an Air Fryer, others will be jealous that they don't have one too! Don't feel left out - get your own today!!!
7) Flavor - That crunchy exterior is something most people crave in their favorite fried foods. The toughest part about air frying is getting that crunchy texture. That's why people prefer deep fryers over Air Fryers. However, if you get it right, it will be crunchy and delicious!
8) Time saver - Cooking with an Air Fryer means you will have more time to do other things in your life! It doesn't take long to make anything in an Air Fryer, and most meals can be made in much less time than they would with a deep fryer.
9) Less mess - There is far less mess when you use an Air Fryer to cook your food. With a deep fryer, there is a lot of oil that is splattered during cooking. With an Air Fryer, there is no grease splattering and it's so easy to clean.

CHAPTER 6:

Help In Choosing the Best Air Fryer on The Market

If you're a fan of fried or oven baked food, but you don't want the high level of unhealthy fats that come from frying them in oil, then an Air Fryer may be just what you need! These cookers have been around since the early 2000s and they gain popularity as more people learn about their benefits.

Ninja Air Fryer Max XL

Ninja Air Fryer Max XL is the best Air Fryer you can buy. A few reasons why it's such an amazing purchase include that it doesn't need any oil, it has a digital timer, and it also has six settings for cooking times and temperatures. With this appliance, there's no excuse for not having fried or seared food in your life anymore!

The Ninja Air Fryer Max XL is sold on Amazon with free shipping. It usually costs around $68. It's a great price for such an awesome product, but with Free Shipping, this Fryer is only $64.99.

The item features six options to cook food. These are: low heat (200 degrees F), medium heat (375 degrees F), high heat (450 degrees F), extra-high temperature (475 degrees F), and slow cook (165-degree F). Although the slow cook option takes around 90 minutes to be fully finished, the other options take only half that time. The Ninja Air Fryer Max XL has a digital timer as well as a removable food tray with all sorts of sizes including 1/4 cup and 1/3 cup.

Ninja Air Fryer Max XL is an amazing appliance for any size kitchen. It works better than any other appliance available out there. The Ninja Air Fryer Max XL is able to bake, fry, steam (can make up to eight different types of foods), make crispy and roasted foods, bake in the oven while it's still warm and more!

GoWise 7-Quart Electric Air Fryer

The GoWise 7-Quart Electric Air Fryer quickly and easily cooks various meals such as French fries, potatoes, wings, and vegetables while giving your food a delicious crispy texture. It's also dishwasher safe for easy cleaning.

The GoWise 7-Quart Electric Air Fryer is not only fashionable but versatile with three customizable cooking settings including turbo mode for added speed or soft mode for cooking slower foods like delicate fruit. Included with the unit are nonstick plates which make cleanup easy.

The 13" x 9" x 12" dimensions of this appliance makes it a perfect fit on any countertop in your kitchen.

The GoWise Electric Air Fryer features an easy-to-read digital display that allows the temperature to be set between 170° F and 400° F, while a built-in timer allows you to cook at different intervals. This unit includes cooking racks so you can prepare a variety of foods at once.

Dash Compact Air Fryer

The Dash Compact Air Fryer is a new kitchen appliance that is designed to be both compact and affordable. It's built with quality in mind, so there are no worries about any breakdowns or malfunctions it will still work as a brand-new machine after years of usage! The cooking surface fits two plates that can hold up to 10 cups of food. There is also a tray on the side which slides out for easy cleaning and maintenance. Another neat feature we love about this Air Fryer is the temperature control you begin at 400 degrees F, but you can regulate it up to 450 degrees F for whatever specific foods you are cooking. Also, the LED light is purposeful and safe to use, so you can see exactly what's going on inside the Air Fryer.

The Dash Compact Air Fryer has a large 12-cup basket to hold your food. It can fit up to ten standard sized pieces of chicken or fish. You also have a four-cup food steamer and a clear lid that covers the entire cooking compartment from top to bottom. The Turbo Defrost feature is there for quick defrosting simply set it at 400 degrees F, and you will be able to defrost frozen items in no time. One of our concerns was that the heating element could get too hot, and it is not a concern with this model.

The Dash Compact Air Fryer is made from BPA-free stainless steel as well as durable materials. You can see the food cooking inside thanks to the see-through top, which adds to the overall satisfaction of the experience because you can see your dinner cooking. The innovative design, as well as the powerful heating element, make it a great air fryer with simple controls.

The package comes with the Dash Compact Air Fryer that measures 17.8 x 11.4 x 13.4 inches in total (with the handle included), as well as a wall mount, instruction manual, and a cookbook full of recipes! It's priced at $149.95 on Amazon, which is a very reasonable price for all you are getting with this Air Fryer.

Philips Compact Air Fryer

Philips Air Fryer is a revolutionary and healthier way of cooking. It uses 80% less oil, cooks food cleaner, and saves money.

This Philips Air Fryer is great for people with little to no kitchen space as it requires only 17 inches of benchtop space. It's also easy to store as it can be simply taken down from the shelf when needed, unlike traditional deep fryers that take up valuable benchtop space and need to be permanently mounted on the wall or in a cupboard below benchtop level.

The Philips Compact Air Fryer has an innovative drop-down basket, which avoids over-crowding and ensures proper air circulation around food for evenly cooked results. It also has a unique draining system, which automatically removes oil from food when it's ready and reduces clean up time.

The two fryer baskets can hold multiple types of food at the same time (e.g., chicken wings, onion rings, and potato wedges) making cooking quicker and easier. The compact design of Philips Air Fryer saves you valuable space in your kitchen and storage is easy, with the basket lifting out for quick cleaning.

The Philips Air Fryer has 3 temperatures to choose from: 180°C, 200°C ad 220°CUP The temperature is automatically set, making it very easy to use. The Philips Air Fryer also has an audible alert system, which sounds when the food is cooked so you don't need to keep checking it and risking getting burnt.

The Philips Air Fryer is not only a healthier alternative to deep frying, it's safer too. Foods are cooked in hot air which removes up to 97% of fat and 100% of cholesterol from the food, making it great for people with heart problems or following a low-fat diet. The Philips Air Fryer offers 16 recipes to get you started from classic fries and chicken wings to sweet desserts and fresh vegetables. Include a little bit of extra virgin olive oil or cooking spray to help the food brown and get that classic delicious taste, texture and crisp.

The Philips Air Fryer is perfect for people with little kitchen space, who love the delicious taste of fried food without the bad effects on their health.

There are also a few things to consider before buying an Air Fryer. The first one is where you'll be using it at. If you're working in a small kitchen, you'll have less space to work with, so keep that in mind when shopping for one. If you're planning on using it outside of the kitchen then you should get something that's portable and lightweight. You should also consider how much use your Air Fryer will be getting, as this can help you decide between certain models out there.

Another thing to think about is what features you want on your Air Fryer, as they do come with extra perks such as timers, automatic shut off functions, interchangeable basket sizes, and more. What you're looking for most will dictate which are the best Air Fryers for you. Also, do make sure to buy an Air Fryer that can be used indoors and not just outdoors, as there are a few models out there that aren't really meant for indoor use.

CHAPTER 7:

Recipes for Breakfast

1. Strawberries Oatmeal

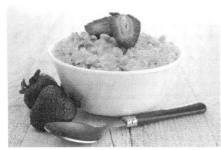

Preparation Time: 5 minutes
Cooking Time: 15 minutes
Servings: 4
Ingredients:
- ½ cup coconut shredded
- ¼ cup strawberries
- 2 cups coconut milk
- ¼ tsp. vanilla extract
- 2 tsp. stevia
- Cooking spray

Directions:
1. Grease the Air Fryer's pan with the cooking spray, add all the ingredients inside, and toss
2. Cook at 365°F for 15 minutes, divide into bowls and serve for breakfast

Nutrition:
- Calories: 142
- Fat: 7g
- Fiber: 2g
- Carbohydrates: 3g
- Protein: 5g

2. Tuna Sandwiches

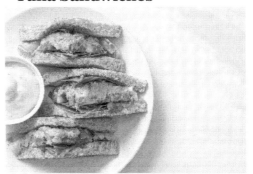

Preparation Time: 10 minutes
Cooking Time: 5 minutes
Servings: 2
Ingredients:
- 16 oz canned tuna, drained
- ¼ cup mayonnaise
- 2 tablespoons mustard
- 1 tablespoon lemon juice
- 2 green onions, chopped
- 3 English muffins, halved
- 3 tablespoons butter
- 6 provolone cheese

Directions:
1. In a bowl, mix tuna with mayo, lemon juice, mustard, and green onions and stir.
2. Grease muffin halves with the butter, place them in the preheated Air Fryer, and bake them at 350°F for 4 minutes.
3. Spread tuna mix on muffin halves, top each with provolone cheese, return sandwiches to Air Fryer and cook them for 4 minutes, divide among plates and serve for breakfast right away. Enjoy!

Nutrition:
- Calories: 182
- Fat: 4g
- Fiber: 7g
- Carbohydrates: 8g
- Protein: 6g

3. Garlic Potatoes with Bacon

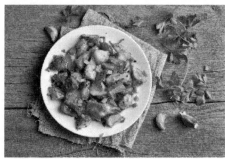

Preparation Time: 10 minutes
Cooking Time: 20 minutes
Servings: 2
Ingredients:

- 4 potatoes, peeled and cut into medium cubes
- 6 garlic cloves, minced
- 4 bacon slices, chopped
- 2 rosemary springs, chopped
- 1 tablespoon olive oil
- Salt and black pepper to the taste
- 2 eggs, whisked

Directions:

1. In your Air Fryer's pan, mix oil with potatoes, garlic, bacon, rosemary, salt, pepper, and eggs and whisk.
2. Cook potatoes at 400 degrees F for 20 minutes, divide everything on plates, and serve for breakfast. Enjoy!

Nutrition:

- Calories: 211 Fat: 3g
- Fiber: 5g
- Carbohydrates: 8g
- Protein: 5g

4. Chicken & Zucchini Omelet

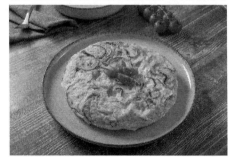

Preparation Time: 15 minutes
Cooking Time: 35 minutes
Servings: 2
Ingredients:

- 8 eggs
- ½ cup milk
- Salt and ground black pepper to taste
- 1 cup cooked chicken, chopped
- 1 cup Cheddar cheese, shredded
- ½ cup fresh chives, chopped
- ¾ cup zucchini, chopped

Directions:

1. In a bowl, add the eggs, milk, salt, and black pepper and beat well. Add the remaining ingredients and stir to combine. Place the mixture into a greased baking pan. Press the "Power Button" of Air Fry Oven and turn the dial to select the "Air Bake" mode.
2. Press the Time button and again turn the dial to set the cooking time to 35 minutes. Now push the Temp button and rotate the dial to set the temperature at 315 degrees F.
3. Press the "Start/Pause" button to start. When the unit beeps to show that it is preheated, open the lid. Arrange pan over the "Wire Rack" and insert in the oven.
4. Cut into equal-sized wedges and serve hot.

Nutrition:

- Calories: 209
- Fat: 13.3 g
- Carbohydrates: 2.3 g
- Fiber: 0.3 g
- Sugar: 1.8 g
- Protein: 9.8 g

5. Tomatoes and Swiss Chard Bake

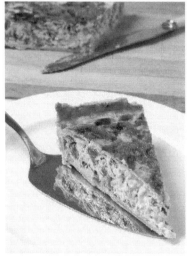

Preparation Time: 5 minutes
Cooking Time: 15 minutes
Servings: 4
Ingredients:

- 4 eggs whisked
- 3 oz. Swiss chard chopped.
- 1 cup tomatoes cubed

- 1 tsp. olive oil
- Salt and black pepper to taste.

Directions:
1. Take a bowl and mix the eggs with the rest of the ingredients except the oil and whisk well.
2. Grease a pan that fits the fryer with the oil, pour the Swiss chard mix, and cook at 359°F for 15 minutes.
3. Divide between plates and serve.

Nutrition:
- Calories: 202 Fat: 14g
- Fiber: 3g
- Carbohydrates: 5g
- Protein: 12g

6. Shrimp Frittata

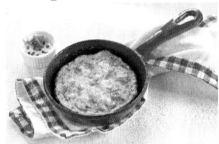

Preparation Time: 10 minutes
Cooking Time: 15 minutes
Servings: 2
Ingredients:
- 4 eggs
- ½ teaspoon basil, dried
- Cooking spray
- Salt and black pepper to the taste
- ½ cup rice, cooked
- ½ cup shrimp, cooked, peeled, deveined, and chopped
- ½ cup baby spinach, chopped
- ½ cup Monterey jack cheese, grated

Directions:
1. In a bowl, mix eggs with salt, pepper, and basil and whisk. Grease your Air Fryer's pan with cooking spray and add rice, shrimp, and spinach. Add eggs mix, sprinkle cheese all over and cook in your Air Fryer at 350 degrees F for 10 minutes.
2. Divide among plates and serve for breakfast. Enjoy!

Nutrition:
- Calories: 162 Fat: 6
- Fiber: 5 Carbohydrates: 8
- Protein: 4

7. Zucchini Fritters

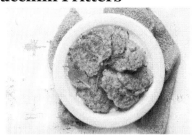

Preparation Time: 15 minutes
Cooking Time: 7 minutes
Servings: 2
Ingredients:
- 10½ oz. zucchini, grated and squeezed
- 7 oz. Halloumi cheese
- ¼ cup all-purpose flour
- 2 eggs
- 1 teaspoon fresh dill, minced
- Salt and ground black pepper, as required

Directions:
1. In a large bowl and mix together all the ingredients.
2. Make a small-sized fritter from the mixture.
3. Press "Power Button" of Air Fry Oven and turn the dial to select the "Air Fry" mode.
4. Press the Time button and again turn the dial to set the cooking time to 7 minutes.
5. Now push the Temp button and rotate the dial to set the temperature at 355°F.
6. Press the "Start/Pause" button to start.
7. When the unit beeps to show that it is preheated, open the lid.
8. Arrange fritters into grease "Sheet Pan" and insert in the oven.
9. Serve warm.

Nutrition:
- Calories: 253
- Fat: 17.2 g
- Carbohydrates: 10 g
- Fiber: 1.1 g
- Sugar: 2.7 g
- Protein: 15.2 g

8. Chicken Omelet

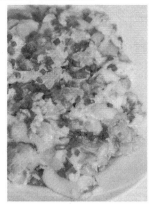

Preparation Time: 10 minutes
Cooking Time: 16 minutes
Servings: 2
Ingredients:

- 1 teaspoon butter
- 1 small yellow onion, chopped
- ½ jalapeño pepper, seeded and chopped
- 3 eggs
- Salt and ground black pepper to taste
- ¼ cup cooked chicken, shredded

Directions:

1. In a frying pan, melt the butter over medium heat and cook the onion for about 4-5 minutes. Add the jalapeño pepper and cook for about 1 minute.
2. Remove from the heat and set aside to cool slightly. Meanwhile, in a bowl, add the eggs, salt, and black pepper and beat well.
3. Add the onion mixture and chicken and stir to combine. Place the chicken mixture into a small baking pan.
4. Press "Power Button" of Air Fry Oven and turn the dial to select the "Air Fry" mode.
5. Press the Time button and again turn the dial to set the cooking time to 6 minutes.
6. Now push the Temp button and rotate the dial to set the temperature at 355°F.
7. Press the "Start/Pause" button to start.
8. When the unit beeps to show that it is preheated, open the lid.
9. Arrange pan over the "Wire Rack" and insert in the oven.
10. Cut the omelet into 2 portions and serve hot.

Nutrition:

- Calories: 153 Fat: 9.1 g
- Carbohydrates: 4 g
- Fiber: 0.9 g Sugar: 2.1 g
- Protein: 13.8 g

9. Scrambled Eggs

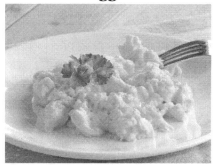

Preparation Time: 5 minutes
Cooking Time: 20 minutes
Servings: 2
Ingredients:

- 4 large eggs.
- ½ cup shredded sharp Cheddar cheese.
- 2 tbsp. unsalted butter melted.

Directions:

1. Crack eggs into a 2-cup round baking dish and whisk.
2. Place dish into the Air Fryer basket.
3. Adjust the temperature to 400°F and set the timer for 10 minutes.
4. After 5 minutes, stir the eggs and add the butter and cheese.
5. Let cook for 3 more minutes and stir again.
6. Allow eggs to finish cooking an additional 2 minutes or remove if they are to your desired liking.
7. Use a fork to fluff. Serve warm.

Nutrition:

- Calories: 359 Protein: 19.5g
- Fiber: 0.0g
- Fat: 27.6g
- Carbohydrates: 1.1g

10. Almond Crust Chicken

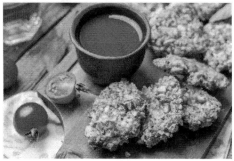

Preparation Time: 10 minutes
Cooking Time: 25 minutes
Servings: 2
Ingredients:

- 2 chicken breasts, skinless and boneless

- 1 tbsp Dijon mustard
- 2 tbsp mayonnaise
- ¼ cup almonds
- Pepper to taste
- Salt to taste

Directions:
1. Add almond into the food processor and process until finely ground.
2. Transfer almonds to a plate and set them aside.
3. Mix mustard and mayonnaise and spread over chicken.
4. Coat chicken with almond and place it into the Air Fryer basket and cook at 350°F for 25 minutes.
5. Serve and enjoy.

Nutrition:
- Calories: 409
- Fat: 22 g
- Carbohydrates: 6 g
- Sugar: 1.5 g
- Protein: 45 g

11. Mushroom Cheese Salad

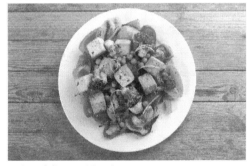

Preparation Time: 10 minutes
Cooking Time: 15 minutes
Servings: 2
Ingredients:
- 10 mushrooms, halved
- 1 tbsp. fresh parsley, chopped
- 1 tbsp. olive oil
- 1 tbsp. mozzarella cheese, grated
- 1 tbsp. cheddar cheese, grated
- 1 tbsp. dried mix herbs
- Pepper to taste
- Salt to taste

Directions:
1. Add all ingredients into the bowl and toss well
2. Transfer bowl mixture into the Air Fryer baking dish
3. Place in the Air Fryer and cook at 380°F for 15 minutes.
4. Serve and enjoy.

Nutrition:
- Calories: 90 Fat: 7 g
- Carbohydrates: 2 g
- Sugar: 1 g
- Protein: 5 g

12. Shrimp Sandwiches

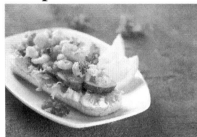

Preparation Time: 10 minutes
Cooking Time: 5 minutes
Servings: 2
Ingredients:
- 1 and ¼ cups cheddar, shredded
- 6 oz canned tiny shrimp, drained
- 3 tablespoons mayonnaise
- 2 tablespoons green onions, chopped
- 4 whole-wheat bread slices
- 2 tablespoons butter, soft

Directions:
1. In a bowl, mix shrimp with cheese, green onion, and mayo, and stir well. Spread this on half of the bread slices, top with the other bread slices, cut into halves diagonally, and spread butter on top.
2. Place sandwiches in your Air Fryer and cook at 350 degrees F for 5 minutes.
3. Divide shrimp sandwiches and serve them for breakfast. Enjoy!

Nutrition:
- Calories: 162
- Fat: 3g
- Fiber: 7g
- Carbohydrates: 12g
- Protein: 4g

13. Mushrooms and Cheese Spread

Preparation Time: 5 minutes
Cooking Time: 20 minutes
Servings: 4
Ingredients:
- ¼ cup mozzarella shredded

- ½ cup coconut cream
- 1 cup white mushrooms
- A pinch of salt and black pepper
- Cooking spray

Directions:
1. Put the mushrooms in your Air Fryer's basket, grease with cooking spray, and cook at 370°F for 20 minutes.
2. Transfer to a blender, add the remaining ingredients, pulse well, divide into bowls and serve as a spread

Nutrition:
- Calories: 202 Fat: 12g
- Fiber: 2g Carbohydrates: 5g Protein: 7g

14. Lemony Raspberries Bowls

Preparation Time: 5 minutes
Cooking Time: 12 minutes
Servings: 2
Ingredients:
- 1 cup raspberries
- 2 tbsp. butter
- 2 tbsp. lemon juice
- 1 tsp. cinnamon powder

Directions:
1. In your Air Fryer, mix all the ingredients, toss, cover, cook at 350°F for 12 minutes, divide into bowls and serve for breakfast

Nutrition:
- Calories: 208 Fat: 6g
- Fiber: 9g
- Carbohydrates: 14g
- Protein: 3g

15. Asparagus Salad

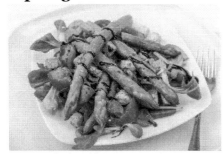

Preparation Time: 5 minutes
Cooking Time: 10 minutes
Servings: 4
Ingredients:
- 1 cup baby arugula
- 1 bunch asparagus trimmed
- 1 tbsp. balsamic vinegar
- 1 tbsp. cheddar cheese grated
- A pinch of salt and black pepper
- Cooking spray

Directions:
1. Put the asparagus in your Air Fryer's basket, grease with cooking spray, season with salt and pepper, and cook at 360°F for 10 minutes.
2. Take a bowl and mix the asparagus with the arugula and the vinegar, toss, divide between plates and serve hot with cheese sprinkled on top

Nutrition:
- Calories: 200 Fat: 5g
- Fiber: 1g
- Carbohydrates: 4g
- Protein: 5g

16. Zucchini Squash Mix

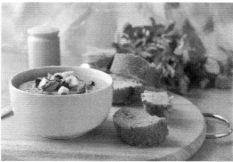

Preparation Time: 10 minutes
Cooking Time: 35 minutes
Servings: 2
Ingredients:
- 1 lb. zucchini, sliced
- 1 tbsp parsley, chopped
- 1 yellow squash, halved, deseeded, and chopped
- 1 tbsp olive oil
- Pepper to taste
- Salt to taste

Directions:
1. Add all ingredients into the large bowl and mix well.
2. Transfer bowl mixture into the Air Fryer basket and cook at 400°F for 35 minutes.
3. Serve and enjoy.

Nutrition:
- Calories: 49
- Fat: 3 g
- Carbohydrates: 4 g
- Sugar: 2 g
- Protein: 1.5 g

17. Bacon-Wrapped Filet Mignon

Preparation Time: 10 minutes
Cooking Time: 15 minutes
Servings: 2
Ingredients:
- 2 bacon slices
- 2 (4-ounce) filet mignon
- Salt and ground black pepper, as required
- Olive oil cooking spray

Directions:
1. Wrap 1 bacon slice around each filet mignon and secure with toothpicks.
2. Season the fillets with salt and black pepper lightly. Arrange the filet mignon onto a cooling rack and spray with cooking spray.
3. Arrange the drip pan in the bottom of the Air Fryer Oven cooking chamber.
4. Select "Air Fry" and then adjust the temperature to 375 degrees F.
5. Set the timer for 15 minutes and press the "Start". When the display shows "Add Food" insert the cooking rack in the center position. When the display shows "Turn Food" turn the filets. When cooking time is complete, remove the rack from Air Fryer oven and serve hot.

Nutrition:
- Calories: 360 Fat: 19.6 g
- Carbohydrates: 0.4 g Protein: 42.6 g

18. Pumpkin Pancakes

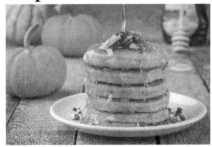

Preparation Time: 15 minutes
Cooking Time: 12 minutes
Servings: 2
Ingredients:
- 1 square puff pastry
- 3 tablespoons pumpkin filling n
- 1 small egg, beaten

Directions:
1. Roll out a square of puff pastry and layer it with pumpkin pie filling, leaving about ¼-inch space around the edges.
2. Cut it up into 8 equal-sized square pieces and coat the edges with a beaten egg.
3. Press "Power Button" of Air Fry Oven and turn the dial to select the "Air Fry" mode. Press the Time button and again turn the dial to set the cooking time to 12 minutes. Now push the Temp button and rotate the dial to set the temperature at 355 degrees F. Press the "Start/Pause" button to start.
4. When the unit beeps to show that it is preheated, open the lid. Arrange the squares into a greased sheet pan and insert them in the oven. Serve warm.

Nutrition:
- Calories: 109 Fat: 6.7 g
- Carbohydrates: 9.8 g
- Fiber: 0.5 g Sugar: 2.6 g Protein: 2.4 g

19. Onion Omelet

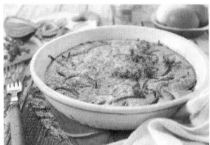

Preparation Time: 10 minutes
Cooking Time: 15 minutes
Servings: 2
Ingredients:
- 4 eggs
- ¼ teaspoon low-sodium soy sauce
- Ground black pepper, as required
- 1 teaspoon butter
- 1 medium yellow onion, sliced
- ¼ cup Cheddar cheese, grated

Directions:
1. In a skillet, melt the butter over medium heat and cook the onion and cook for about 8-10 minutes.
2. Remove from the heat and set aside to cool slightly.
3. Meanwhile, in a bowl, add the eggs, soy sauce, and black pepper and beat well.
4. Add the cooked onion and gently, stir to combine.
5. Place the zucchini mixture into a small baking pan. Press "Power Button" of Air Fry Oven and turn the dial to select the "Air Fry" mode.
6. Press the Time button and again turn the dial to set the cooking time to 5 minutes.

7. Now push the Temp button and rotate the dial to set the temperature at 355 degrees F. Press the "Start/Pause" button to start.
8. When the unit beeps to show that it is preheated, open the lid.
9. Arrange the pan over the "Wire Rack" and insert it in the oven.
10. Cut the omelet into 2 portions and serve hot.

Nutrition:
- Calories: 222 Carbohydrates: 6.1 g
- Fiber: 1.2 g Sugar: 3.1 g
- Protein: 15.3 g

20. Sweetened Breakfast Oats

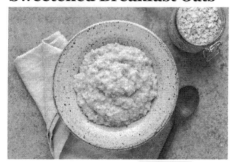

Preparation Time: 10 minutes
Cooking Time: 7 minutes
Servings: 4
Ingredients:
- 1 cup steel-cut oats
- 3/4 cup shredded coconut
- 1/4 tsp ground ginger
- 1/4 tsp ground nutmeg
- 1/2 tsp ground cinnamon
- 1/4 cup raisins
- 1 large apple, chopped
- 2 large carrots, grated
- 1 cup of coconut milk
- 3 cups of water

Directions:
1. Add oats, nutmeg, ginger, cinnamon, raisins, apple, carrots, milk, and water into the instant pot and stir to combine.
2. Seal pot with lid and cook on manual mode for 4 minutes.
3. Once done then allow to release pressure naturally for 20 minutes then release using the quick-release method. Open the lid.
4. Top with coconut and serve.

Nutrition:
- Calories: 341 Fat: 20.8 g
- Carbohydrates: 38.2 g
- Sugar: 16.1 g Protein: 5.3 g

21. Veggie Quiche Muffins

Preparation Time: 20 minutes
Cooking Time: 15 minutes
Servings: 1
Ingredients:
- ¾ cup Shredded cheddar
- 1 cup green onion
- 1 cup Chopped broccoli
- 1 cup diced tomatoes
- 2 cups milk
- 4 eggs
- 1 cup Pancake mix
- 1 tsp. oregano
- ½ tsp. salt
- ½ tsp. pepper

Directions:
1. Set oven to 375°F, and lightly grease a 12-cup muffin tin with oil.
2. Sprinkle tomatoes, broccoli, onions, and cheddar into muffin cups.
3. Combine remaining ingredients in a medium bowl, whisk to combine then pour evenly on top of veggies.
4. Set to bake in preheated oven for about 40 min or until golden brown.
5. Allow cooling slightly (about 5 min) then servings. Enjoy!

Nutrition:
- Calories: 59 Carbohydrates: 2.9 g
- Protein: 5.1 g
- Fat: 3.2g

22. Steel Cut Oat Blueberry Pancakes

Preparation Time: 10 minutes
Cooking Time: 10 minutes
Servings: 1
Ingredients:
- 1½ cup water
- ½ cup oats
- 1/8 tsp. salt
- 1 cup flour
- ½ tsp. baking powder
- ½ tsp. baking soda
- 1 egg
- 1 cup milk ½ cup Greek yogurt
- 1 cup Frozen blueberries
- ¾ cup agave nectar

Directions:
1. Combine oats, salt, and water together in a medium saucepan, stir, and allow to come to a boil over high heat.
2. Set it to low and simmer for 10 min, or until oats are tender. Set aside.
3. Combine all remaining ingredients, except agave nectar, in a medium bowl, then fold in oats.
4. Preheat griddle and lightly grease. Cook ¼ cup of batter at a time for about 3 min per side. Garnish with agave.

Nutrition:
- Calories: 257 Carbohydrates: 46 g
- Protein: 14 g Fat: 7 g

23. Very Berry Muesli

Preparation Time: 2 hours
Cooking Time: 2 hours
Servings: 1

Ingredients:
- 1 cup oats
- 1 cup fruit-flavored yogurt
- ½ cup Milk
- 1/8 tsp. Salt
- ½ cup Dried raisins
- ½ cup Chopped apple
- ½ cup Frozen blueberries
- ¼ cup Chopped walnuts

Directions:
1. Combine yogurt, salt, and oats in a medium bowl, mix well, then cover the mixture tightly.
2. Place in the refrigerator to cool for 6 hours.
3. Add raisins, and apples the gently fold.
4. Top with walnuts and servings. Enjoy!

Nutrition:
- Calories: 198 Carbohydrates: 31.2 g
- Protein: 6 g Fat: 4.3 g

24. Strawberry & Mushroom Breakfast Sandwich

Preparation Time: 5 min
Cooking Time: 5 min
Servings: 1

Ingredients:
- 8 oz. Cream cheese
- 1 tbsp. Honey
- 1 tbsp. Grated lemon zest
- 4 sliced portobello mushrooms
- 2 cup Sliced strawberries

Directions:
1. Add honey, lemon zest, and cheese to a food processor, and process until fully incorporated.
2. Use cheese mixture to spread on mushrooms as you would butter.
3. Top with strawberries. Enjoy!

Nutrition:
- Calories: 180 Carbohydrates: 6 g
- Protein: 2 g Fat: 16 g

25. Shakshuka Egg Bake

Preparation Time: 10 minutes
Cooking Time: 15 minutes
Servings: 1

Ingredients:
- 1 teaspoon extra-virgin olive oil
- ½ onion, minced
- 1 garlic clove, minced
- ½ teaspoon smoked paprika
- ½ teaspoon ground cumin
- 1 (15-ounce) can diced tomatoes
- 2 oz. feta cheese, crumbled
- 4 large eggs

Directions:
1. Preheat the oven to 350°F.
2. In a medium skillet over medium heat, heat the oil. Add the onions and garlic, and sauté until translucent, about 5 min. Add the paprika and cumin, and cook a minute longer.
3. Stir in the tomatoes until well combined. Simmer until some of their liquid has evaporated and the mixture begins to thicken to form a sauce, 5 to 10 min.
4. Divide the sauce evenly among 4 ramekins, and repeat with the cheese, sprinkling evenly across.
5. Using a spoon, create wells in the tomato sauce and crack an egg over each, being careful to keep the yolk intact.
6. Bake in the ramekins for 15 min, until the yolk is done to your liking, longer if you like a hard-cooked yolk, and servings. (If you do not have ramekins, crack the eggs into spoon-made wells in the pan and let cook for 5 to 10 min, or per your preference.)

Nutrition:
- Calories: 144 Carbohydrates: 7 g
- Protein: 9 g Fat: 9 g
- Fiber: 1 g Sodium: 455 mg

26. Ricotta Baked in the Oven

Preparation Time: 10 minutes
Cooking Time: 15 minutes
Servings: 1
Ingredients:

- ¼ cup parmesan cheese (grated)
- ½ cup ricotta cheese (low fat)
- 1 teaspoon Dijon mustard
- 1 teaspoon thyme (ground)
- ¼ cup cheddar cheese (shredded)
- 1 egg

Directions:

1. Heat the oven to a temperature of 400°F.
2. Put all the ingredients in one bowl. Stir and mix them well. The mixture will appear to be gritty and slightly brown. But it must be smooth.
3. Use one cookie scoop and divide the mixture into 4 wells of the muffin pan. You can use muffin pans made of silicone as you can use them easily and clean them quickly.
4. Bake it for about 20 min. Then remove from the oven and let it cool a bit. It is ready to be servings.

Nutrition:

- Calories: 190
- Carbohydrates: 4 g
- Protein: 8 g
- Fat: 4 g

27. Poached Eggs Italian Style

Preparation Time: 10 minutes
Cooking Time: 10 minutes
Servings: 2
Ingredients:

- 3 to 4 pieces of jarred red pepper (roasted and sliced)
- 16 oz. of marinara sauce (with the lowest level of sugar)
- 4 eggs
- 4 leaves of fresh basil
- 1 pinch of salt
- 1 pinch of pepper

Directions:

1. Heat a big, rimmed skillet on medium heat. Put the marinara sauce. Then add the red peppers. Crack the eggs one by one making a "well" with the back of one spoon. Sprinkle pepper and salt.
2. Allow it to cook till the eggs become firm or for around 12 min. If you'd like you can put the lid for 2 min at the end.
3. Remove from the heat. Sprinkle basil and **Servings:** in a bowl or plate.

Nutrition:

- Calories: 110
- Carbohydrates: 7 g
- Protein: 8 g
- Fat: 6 g

28. Denver Egg Muffins with Ham Crust

Preparation Time: 15 minutes
Cooking Time: 15 minutes
Servings: 1
Ingredients:

- Nonstick cooking time spray
- 12 slices deli ham
- ½ cup cheddar cheese
- 1 teaspoon extra-virgin olive oil
- ½ onion, diced
- ½ green pepper, minced
- 10 large eggs
- ¼ cup low-fat milk

Directions:

1. Preheat the oven to 350°F.
2. Grease a 12-compartment muffin tin with cooking time spray.
3. Line each cup with a ham slice, pushing it down to fit tightly against the edge of the well.
4. In a small skillet over medium heat, heat the oil. Add the onion and green pepper, and sauté for 3 min, or until soft. Remove from the heat, and drain any liquid from the pan.
5. In a large bowl, whisk the eggs and milk. Add the cheese and cooked vegetables, and whisk again.
6. Ladle ¼ cup of the egg mixture into each cup. If there is any left over, divide evenly among the cups.
7. Bake for 20 to 25 min, or just until the eggs are firm and no longer runny, and servings.

Nutrition:

- Calories: 99
- Carbohydrates: 1 g
- Protein: 8 g
- Fat: 6 g
- Sugars: 1 g
- Sodium: 206 mg

29. Cheesy Slow Cooker Egg Casserole

Preparation Time: 15 min
Cooking Time: 2 hours
Servings: 1
Ingredients:

- 1-pound fresh Italian chicken sausage
- Nonstick cooking time spray
- 1 (30-ounce) bag frozen hash browns
- 1 medium red bell pepper, seeded and diced
- ½ medium onion, diced
- 1 (4-ounce) can mild diced green chiles
- 1½ cup low-fat shredded cheddar cheese, divided into three, ½-cup servings
- 12 large eggs
- 1 cup low-fat milk
- ½ teaspoon salt
- ½ teaspoon freshly ground black pepper

Directions:

1. Remove the casings from the sausage, and discard.
2. In a large skillet over medium heat, brown the meat, breaking it into smaller pieces as it cooks, about 7 min, or until no longer pink.
3. Spray a 5-quart slow cooker with nonstick cooking time spray, and layer half of the frozen hash browns, cooked sausage, pepper, onion, and chiles, plus ½ cup of cheese. Repeat with the remaining hash browns, sausage, pepper, onion, and chiles, plus another ½ cup of cheese.
4. In a large bowl, whisk the eggs, milk, salt, and pepper.
5. Pour the egg mixture over the potato-sausage layers, and top with the remaining ½ cup of cheese.
6. Cook on high for 4 hours or on low for 8 hours, and servings.

Nutrition:

- Calories: 348 Carbohydrates: 24 g
- Protein: 27 g Fat: 17 g
- Sugars: 3 g Sodium: 783 mg

30. Make-Ahead Breakfast Burritos

Preparation Time: 15 minutes
Cooking Time: 20 minutes
Servings: 1
Ingredients:

- 12 large eggs
- ¼ cup low-fat milk
- 1 teaspoon extra-virgin olive oil
- ½ medium yellow onion, diced
- 1 medium green bell pepper, seeded and diced
- 1 cup canned black beans, drained and rinsed
- 8 (7- to 8-inch) whole wheat tortillas
- ½ cup shredded cheddar cheese
- 8 oz salsa

Directions:

1. In a large bowl, whisk together the eggs and milk.
2. In a large skillet over medium heat, heat the oil. Add the onion, bell pepper, and black beans. Sauté until the onion is translucent, about 5 min, and transfer to a plate.
3. Pour the egg mixture into the skillet, and gently stir until the eggs are fluffy and firm. Remove from the heat.
4. Divide the eggs and onion mixture evenly among the tortillas, and top with the cheese and salsa.
5. With both sides of the first tortilla tucked in, roll tightly to close. Repeat with the remaining tortillas.
6. Serving immediately, or freeze for up to 3 months. If freezing, wrap the burritos in paper towels and cover tightly with aluminum foil for storage.

Nutrition:

- Calories: 264
- Carbohydrates: 24 g
- Protein: 21 g
- Fat: 12 g
- Sugars: 3 g
- Sodium: 593 mg

31. Magic Hot Cereal

Preparation Time: 5 minutes
Cooking Time: 5 minutes
Servings: 1
Ingredients:

- 3/4 cup water
- ¼ cup Bob's Red Mill 7 Grain Hot Cereal
- ¼ teaspoon orange rind, finely grated
- 1 dash kosher salt
- 1 dash ground cinnamon
- 1 pinch fresh ground nutmeg
- 4-5 tablespoons vanilla soy milk

- 2 drops vanilla extract
- 1 teaspoon butter
- 2 tablespoons maple syrup

Directions:
1. In a small pot, add the orange rind to water and bring to a boil.
2. Add cereal, salt, cinnamon, and nutmeg and reduce heat. Stir while cooking and add the soy milk a tablespoon at a time when the liquid has been fully absorbed by the cereal.
3. When the cereal is done, about 6 minutes, add vanilla extract, butter, and maple syrup. Stir to mix and serve hot.

Nutrition:
- Calories: 265 Carbohydrates: 39.7 g
- Protein: 12.5 g Fat: 8.5 g

32. Baked Broccoli and Eggs

Preparation Time: 10 minutes
Cooking Time: 15 minutes
Servings: 1
Ingredients:
- 4 oz. Margarine, light
- 10 oz. Broccoli, frozen, thawed, chopped
- 4 oz. Pimento, jarred, chopped
- 6 tbsps. Flour
- 1 dash Black pepper, freshly ground
- ½ cup Mushrooms, sliced, fresh
- 6 pieces Eggs, large
- ½ pound Cheddar cheese, low fat
- 2 pounds Cottage cheese, nonfat
- 1 teaspoon salt
- 1 dash Paprika

Directions:
1. Set the oven to 350°F to preheat.
2. Meanwhile, place the eggs, broccoli, and all other ingredients in a large bowl. Stir to combine.
3. Use cooking time spray to coat the sides and bottom of a casserole dish (2-quart).
4. Fill the preparation time dish with the broccoli-egg mixture, making sure to spread it evenly.
5. Bake in the oven for one hour and thirty min.
6. Serve immediately.

Nutrition:
- Calories: 129 Carbohydrates: 2 g
- Protein: 10 g Fat: 9 g
- Sugars: 2 g Sodium: 218 mg

33. Broccoli and Tofu Quiche

Preparation Time: 10 minutes
Cooking Time: 15 minutes
Servings: 1
Ingredients:
- ¼ Teaspoon salt
- ¼ pound mushrooms, chopped
- 1 tbsp. Pickled plum/ white miso paste
- 1-piece yellow onion, chopped
- 2 tbsps. Sesame tahini
- ½ cup bulgur wheat, uncooked
- 1 tbsp. Sesame oil
- ½ pound broccoli, chopped
- 1 ½ pounds tofu
- 1 tbsp. Tamari

Directions:
1. Set the oven at 350°F to preheat.
2. Fill a small pot with water (1 cup) and heat on medium. Bring to a boil before adding in the bulgur and salt.
3. Stir to combine and allow the mixture to boil again. Reduce heat to low and cover to cook for about fifteen min. Meanwhile, grease a pie pan (9-inch) with a little oil. Pour the cooked bulgur into the pie pan, pressing lightly to spread it evenly at the bottom. Place in the oven to bake for about twelve min or until crusty on top. Let stand to cool.
4. Heat a large skillet (nonstick) on medium-high before adding the onions. Stir in the mushrooms and broccoli and cook for two min. Cover and immediately remove from heat. Meanwhile, fill the food processor with the tofu. Add the tamari, tahini, and umeboshi paste. Process until well-combined and smooth, then pour into a large bowl.
5. Add the cooked veggies and gently toss until evenly coated. Transfer the veggie mixture onto the crusted bulgur. Bake in the oven for about half an hour. Once done, let stand on a wire rack. After ten min, slice into 6 portions and serve immediately.

Nutrition:
- Calories: 248
- Carbohydrates: 27.2 g
- Protein: 30.6 g
- Fat: 3.6 g
- Sodium: 718 mg

34. Cheese-Filled Acorn Squash

Preparation Time: 10 minutes
Cooking Time: 50 minutes
Servings: 1
Ingredients:

- 1 pound tofu, firm
- 1 teaspoon basil
- 1 pinch black pepper, freshly ground
- 1 teaspoon onion, chopped finely
- 1 teaspoon garlic powder
- 1 cup cheddar cheese, reduced fat, shredded
- 2 pieces acorn squash, halved, seeded
- 1 cup celery, diced
- 1 cup mushrooms, fresh, sliced
- 1 teaspoon oregano
- 1/8 teaspoon salt
- 8 oz. tomato sauce

Directions:

1. Set the oven at 350°F to preheat.
2. Arrange the acorn squash pieces, with their cut sides facing down, at the bottom of a glass dish.
3. Place in the microwave oven and cook for about twenty min or until softened. Set aside.
4. Heat a saucepan (nonstick) on medium, then add the tofu (sliced into cubes). Cook until browned before stirring in the onion and celery. Cook for two min or until the onion is translucent.
5. Add the mushrooms. Stir to combine and cook for an additional two to three min. Pour in the tomato sauce as well as the dry seasonings.
6. Give everything a good stir, then spoon equal portions of the mixture inside the acorn squash pieces.
7. Cover and place in the oven to cook for about fifteen min. Uncover and top with the cheese before returning to the oven. Cook for five more min or until the cheese is melted and bubbling.
8. **Servings:** immediately.

Nutrition:

- Calories: 328
- Carbohydrates: 47.5 g
- Protein: 16.9 g
- Fat: 10.8 g
- Sodium: 557 mg

35. Cheesy Spinach Bake

Preparation Time: 5 minutes
Cooking Time: 35 minutes
Servings: 1
Ingredients:

- 2 pieces eggs, whole
- ½ cup parmesan cheese
- 2 cups cottage cheese, fat-free/ low fat
- 10 oz. spinach, frozen, thawed, drained

Directions:

1. Set the oven to 350°F to preheat. Meanwhile, line a baking pan (8x8) with parchment paper.
2. Place all ingredients in a large bowl. Stir to combine. Pour the cheesy spinach mixture into the preparation time bed pan. Place in the oven to bake for twenty to thirty min or until the cheese on top is bubbling.
3. Remove from the oven and allow to cool for five min.
4. Serve sprinkled with garlic, salt, and pepper. Enjoy.

Nutrition:

- Calories: 292 Carbohydrates: 4.5 g
- Protein: 26 g Fat: 19 g
- Sodium: 735 mg

36. Greek Yogurt, Granola, and Berry Parfait

Preparation Time: 10 minutes
Cooking Time: 15 minutes or less
Servings: 1
Ingredients:

- ½ cup nonfat plain Greek yogurt
- 1 tbsp. rolled oats
- ¼ cup fresh blueberries
- ¼ cup fresh raspberries
- 1 tbsp. chopped walnuts
- 1 tbsp. chopped pecans
- 1 teaspoon honey

Directions:

1. Place the yogurt in a 6-ounce glass.
2. Top with oats, blueberries, raspberries, walnuts, and pecans. Drizzle the honey on top. Enjoy immediately.

Nutrition:

- Calories: 245 Carbohydrates: 25 g
- Protein: 16 g Fat: 11 g
- Sugars: 21 g Sodium: 46 mg

37. Eggs Florentine

Preparation Time: 10 minutes
Cooking Time: 10 minutes
Servings: 1
Ingredients:

- 2 large eggs
- 1 tbsp. Extra virgin olive oil (unfiltered)
- 5 tbsps. Egg fast Alfredo sauce
- 1 tbsp. Organic parmigiana Reggiano wedge (divided)
- 3 g Organic baby spinach
- 1 pinch red pepper flakes

Directions:

1. Set oven rack in the top groove nearest to the broiler. Set broiler to preheat.
2. Place olive oil in a non-stick skillet and put to heat over medium-high heat.
3. Gently, fry eggs over medium flame, until egg whites are opaque but the yolk is still runny. This takes roughly 4 min. Do not turn over eggs.
4. Preparation time casserole in the meantime. Dribble some olive oil in each casserole container or spray with cooking time spray (olive oil).
5. In the bottom of the casserole, spread half of the Alfredo sauce. Slide gently, the half-done egg atop sauce.
6. Spread leftover Alfredo sauce and half of the parmesan cheese over eggs.
7. Set casserole under the broiler and broil for 2-3 min or until the eggs have formed and the top has bubbly golden spots.
8. Remove from broiler and top with thinly sliced (julienne) baby spinach leaves, unused parmesan cheese, and a dash of red pepper flakes.
9. Serve instantly.

Nutrition:

- Calories: 529
- Carbohydrates: 3 g
- Protein: 29 g
- Fat: 3 g

38. Mexican Scrambled Eggs

Preparation Time: 10 minutes
Cooking Time: 5 minutes
Servings: 1
Ingredients:

- 6 eggs (lightly beaten)
- 1 tomato (diced)
- 3 oz. cheese (shredded)
- 1 tbsp. butter (for frying)

Directions:

1. Set a large skillet with butter over medium heat and allow it to melt.
2. Add tomatoes and green onions then cook, while stirring, until fragrant (about 3 min).
3. Add eggs, and continue to cook, while stirring, until almost set (about 2 min).
4. Add cheese, and season to taste continue cooking time until the cheese melts (about another minute).
5. Serve and enjoy.

Nutrition:

- Calories: 239
- Carbohydrates: 1 g
- Protein: 8 g
- Fat: 3.7 g

39. Spinach Omelet

Preparation Time: 10 min
Cooking Time: 10 min
Servings: 1
Ingredients:

- 2 tbsp olive oil
- 1 cup spinach, chopped
- 1 cup Swiss chard, chopped
- 3 eggs 1 tsp garlic powder
- ½ tsp sea salt ¼ tsp red pepper flakes

Directions:

1. Grease the pressure cooker's bottom with 2 tablespoons of olive oil.
2. Press the beans/lentils button and add greens. Stir-fry for 5 min. Remove from the cooker and set aside.
3. Whisk together eggs, garlic powder, salt, and red pepper flakes. Pour the mixture into the stainless-steel insert.
4. Spread the eggs evenly with a wooden spatula and cook for about 2-3 min.
5. Using a spatula, ease around the edges and slide to a **Servings:** plate. Add greens and fold it over in half.

Nutrition:

- Calories: 227
- Carbohydrates: 2.3 g
- Protein: 20 g
- Fat: 3 g

40. Egg and Avocado Toast

Preparation Time: 5 minutes
Cooking Time: 5 minutes
Servings: 1
Ingredients:

- 1 slice whole-grain bread
- 1 teaspoon Dijon mustard
- ¼ avocado, peeled, pitted, and sliced
- 1 hard-boiled egg, cut into slices
- 1 tablespoon chopped fresh cilantro
- Freshly ground black pepper (optional)

Directions:

1. Toast the bread.
2. Spread the mustard over the toast then top with the avocado slices.
3. Layer the egg slices on top. Sprinkle with cilantro, season with pepper (if using) to taste, and enjoy.
4. POST-OP TIP: Bread can be filling. I suggest waiting until you are at least six months post-op before adding it to your weekly breakfast rotation. Eat slowly, chew well, and stop when you feel full.

Nutrition:

- Calories: 239 Carbohydrates: 22 g
- Protein: 12 g Fat: 12 g
- Sugars: 3 g Sodium: 334 mg

CHAPTER 8:

Recipes for Lunch

41. Easy Rosemary Lamb Chops

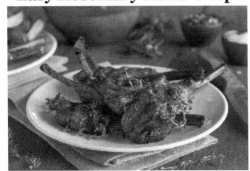

Preparation Time: 10 minutes
Cooking Time: 6 minutes
Servings: 4
Ingredients:

- 4 lamb chops
- 2 tbsps. dried rosemary
- ¼ cup fresh lemon juice
- Pepper to taste
- Salt to taste

Directions:
1. In a medium bowl, mix lemon juice, rosemary, pepper, and salt. Brush lemon juice rosemary mixture over lamb chops.
2. Place lamb chops on Air Fryer oven tray and air fry at 400°F for 3 minutes. Turn lamb chops to the other side and cook for 3 minutes more. Serve and enjoy.

Nutrition:
- Calories: 267
- Fat: 21.7 g.
- Carbohydrates 1.4 g.
- Protein: 16.9 g.

42. Greek Lamb Chops

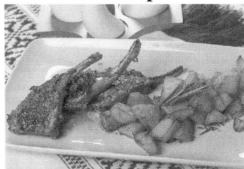

Preparation Time: 10 minutes
Cooking Time: 10 minutes
Servings: 4
Ingredients:

- 2 lbs. lamb chops
- 2 tsps. garlic, minced
- 1 ½ tsp. dried oregano
- ¼ cup fresh lemon juice
- ¼ cup olive oil
- ½ tsp. pepper
- 1 tsp. salt

Directions:
1. Add lamb chops in a mixing bowl. Add the remaining ingredients over the lamb chops and coat well.
2. Arrange lamb chops on the Air Fryer oven tray and cook at 400°F for 5 minutes.
3. Turn lamb chops and cook for 5 minutes more.
4. Serve and enjoy.

Nutrition:
- Calories: 538
- Fat: 29.4 g.
- Carbohydrates 1.3 g.
- Protein: 64 g.

43. Easy Beef Roast

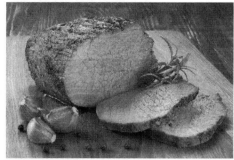

Preparation Time: 10 minutes
Cooking Time: 45 minutes
Servings: 6
Ingredients:

- 2 ½ lbs. beef roast
- 2 tbsps. Italian seasoning

Directions:
1. Arrange roast on the rotisserie spite.
2. Rub roast with Italian seasoning then insert into the Instant Vortex Air Fryer Oven.
3. Air fry at 350°F for 45 minutes or until the internal temperature of the roast reaches 145°F.
4. Slice and serve.

Nutrition:
- Calories: 365 Fat: 13.2 g.
- Carbohydrates 0.5 g.
- Protein: 57.4 g.

44. Juicy Pork Chops

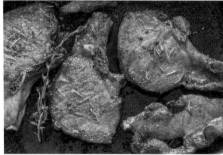

Preparation Time: 10 minutes
Cooking Time: 16 minutes
Servings: 4
Ingredients:

- 4 pork chops, boneless
- 2 tsps. olive oil
- ½ tsp. celery seed
- ½ tsp. parsley
- ½ tsp. granulated onion
- ½ tsp. granulated garlic
- ¼ tsp. sugar
- ½ tsp. salt

Directions:
1. In a small bowl, mix oil, celery seed, parsley, granulated onion, granulated garlic, sugar, and salt.
2. Rub seasoning mixture all over the pork chops.
3. Place pork chops on the Air Fryer oven pan and cook at 350°F for 8 minutes.
4. Turn pork chops to the other side and cook for 8 minutes more.
5. Serve and enjoy.

Nutrition:
- Calories: 279
- Fat: 22.3 g.
- Carbohydrates 0.6 g.
- Protein: 18.1 g.

45. Tuna and Spring Onions Salad

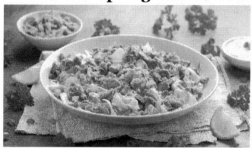

Preparation Time: 5 minutes
Cooking Time: 15 minutes
Servings: 4
Ingredients:

- 14 oz. canned tuna, drained and flaked
- 2 spring onions chopped
- 1 cup arugula
- 1 tbsp. olive oil
- A pinch of salt and black pepper

Directions:
1. In a media bowl, add all ingredients except the oil and arugula and whisk.
2. Preheat the Air Fryer over 360°F, add oil, and grease it. Pour the tuna mix, stir well and cook for 15 minutes.
3. In a salad bowl, combine the arugula with the tuna mix, toss and serve.

Nutrition:
- Calories: 212
- Fat: 8 g.
- Fiber: 3 g.
- Carbohydrates: 5 g.
- Protein: 8 g.

46. Bacon-Wrapped Filet Mignon

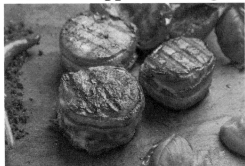

Preparation Time: 10 minutes
Cooking Time: 15 minutes
Servings: 2
Ingredients:

- 2 bacon slices
- 2 (4 oz.) fillet mignon
- Salt and ground black pepper, as required
- Olive oil cooking spray

Directions:

1. Wrap 1 bacon slice around each fillet mignon and secure with toothpicks.
2. Season the fillets with salt and black pepper lightly.
3. Arrange the fillet mignon onto a cooking rack and spray with cooking spray.
4. Place the drip pan in the cooking chamber of the Instant Vortex Plus Air Fryer Oven.
5. Choose "Air Fry" and set the temperature to 375°F.
6. Press the "Start" button after setting the timer for 15 minutes.
7. Place the frying rack in the center position when the display says "Add Food."
8. When the display shows "Turn Food" turn the fillets.
9. When cooking time is complete, remove the rack from Vortex and serve hot.

Nutrition:

- Calories: 360
- Fat: 19.6 g.
- Carbohydrates 0.4 g.
- Protein: 42.6 g.

47. Classic Beef Jerky

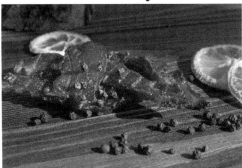

Preparation Time: 10 minutes
Cooking Time: 4 hours
Servings: 4
Ingredients:

- 2 lbs. London broil, sliced thinly
- 1 tsp. onion powder
- 3 tbsps. brown sugar
- 3 tbsps. soy sauce
- 1 tsp. olive oil
- ¾ tsp. garlic powder

Directions:

1. Add all ingredients except meat in the large zip-lock bag.
2. Mix until well combined. Add meat to the bag.
3. Seal bag and massage gently to cover the meat with marinade.
4. Let marinate the meat for 1 hour.
5. Arrange marinated meat slices on an Instant Vortex Air Fryer Tray and dehydrate at 160°F for 4 hours.

Nutrition:

- Calories: 133
- Fat: 4.7 g.
- Carbohydrates 9.4 g.
- Protein: 13.4 g.

48. Flavorful Steak

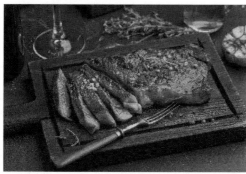

Preparation Time: 10 minutes
Cooking Time: 18 minutes
Servings: 2
Ingredients:

- 2 steaks, rinsed and pat dry
- ½ tsp. garlic powder
- 1 tsp. olive oil
- Pepper to taste
- Salt to taste

Directions:

1. Rub steaks with olive oil and season with garlic powder, pepper, and salt.
2. Preheat the Instant Vortex Air Fryer Oven to 400°F.
3. Place steaks on Air Fryer oven pan and air fry for 10–18 minutes turning halfway through.
4. Serve and enjoy.

Nutrition:

- Calories: 361 Fat: 10.9 g.
- Carbohydrates 0.5 g. Protein: 61.6 g.

49. BBQ Pork Chops

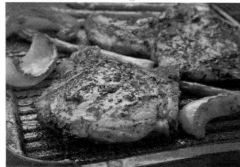

Preparation Time: 10 minutes
Cooking Time: 7 minutes
Servings: 4
Ingredients:

- 4 pork chops

For the rub:

- ½ tsp. allspice
- ½ tsp. dry mustard
- 1 tsp. ground cumin
- 1 tsp. garlic powder
- ½ tsp. chili powder
- ½ tsp. paprika
- 1 tbsp. brown sugar
- 1 tsp. salt

Directions:

1. In a small bowl, mix all rub ingredients and rub all over pork chops.
2. Arrange pork chops on Air Fryer tray and air fry at 400°F for 5 minutes.
3. Turn pork chops to the other side and air fry for 2 minutes more.
4. Serve and enjoy.

Nutrition:

- Calories: 273 Fat: 20.2 g.
- Carbohydrates 3.4 g.
- Protein: 18.4 g.

50. Crispy Meatballs

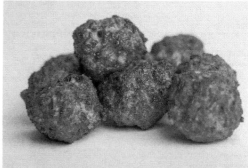

Preparation Time: 10 minutes
Cooking Time: 12 minutes
Servings: 8
Ingredients:

- 1 lb. ground pork
- 1 lb. ground beef
- 1 tbsp. Worcestershire sauce
- ½ cup feta cheese, crumbled
- ½ cup breadcrumbs
- 2 eggs, lightly beaten
- ¼ cup fresh parsley, chopped
- 1 tbsp. garlic, minced
- 1 onion, chopped
- ¼ tsp. pepper
- 1 tsp. salt

Directions:

1. Add all ingredients into the mixing bowl and mix until well combined.
2. Spray Air Fryer oven tray pan with cooking spray.

3. Make small balls from the meat mixture and arrange them on a pan and air fry at 400°F for 10–12 minutes.
4. Serve and enjoy.

Nutrition:
- Calories: 263
- Fat: 9 g.
- Carbohydrates 7.5 g.
- Protein: 35.9 g.

51. Juicy Steak Bites

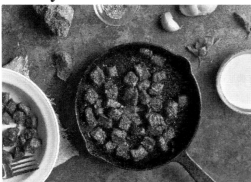

Preparation Time: 10 minutes
Cooking Time: 9 minutes
Servings: 4
Ingredients:
- 1 lb. sirloin steak, cut into bite-size pieces
- 1 tbsp. steak seasoning
- 1 tbsp. olive oil
- Pepper to taste
- Salt to taste

Directions:
1. Preheat the Instant Vortex Air Fryer Oven to 390°F.
2. Add steak pieces into the large mixing bowl. Add steak seasoning, oil, pepper, and salt over steak pieces and toss until well coated.
3. Transfer steak pieces on instant vortex Air Fryer pan and air fry for 5 minutes.
4. Turn steak pieces to the other side and cook for 4 minutes more.
5. Serve and enjoy.

Nutrition:
- Calories: 241
- Fat: 10.6 g.
- Carbohydrates 0 g.
- Protein: 34.4 g.

52. Lemon Garlic Lamb Chops

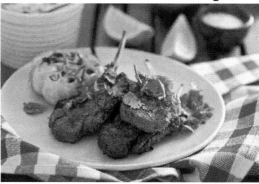

Preparation Time: 10 minutes
Cooking Time: 6 minutes
Servings: 6
Ingredients:
- 6 lamb loin chops
- 2 tbsps. fresh lemon juice
- 1 ½ tbsp. lemon zest
- 1 tbsp. dried rosemary
- 1 tbsp. olive oil
- 1 tbsp. garlic, minced
- Pepper to taste
- Salt to taste

Directions:
1. Add lamb chops in a mixing bowl. Add the remaining ingredients on top of lamb chops and coat well.
2. Arrange lamb chops on Air Fryer oven tray and air fry at 400°F for 3 minutes. Turn lamb chops to another side and air fry for 3 minutes more. Serve and enjoy.

Nutrition:
- Calories: 69
- Fat: 6 g.
- Carbohydrates 1.2 g.
- Protein: 3 g.

53. BBQ Pork Ribs

Preparation Time: 10 minutes
Cooking Time: 12 minutes
Servings: 6
Ingredients:
- 1 slab baby back pork ribs, cut into pieces
- ½ cup BBQ sauce
- ½ tsp. paprika
- Salt to taste

Directions:
1. Add pork ribs to a mixing bowl. Add BBQ sauce, paprika, and salt over pork ribs and coat well, and set aside for 30 minutes.

2. Preheat the Instant Vortex Air Fryer Oven to 350°F.
3. Arrange marinated pork ribs on Instant Vortex Air Fryer Oven pan and cook for 10–12 minutes. Turn halfway through.
4. Serve and enjoy.

Nutrition:
- Calories: 145 Fat: 7 g.
- Carbohydrates 10 g.
- Protein: 9 g.

54. Herb Butter Rib-Eye Steak

Preparation Time: 10 minutes
Cooking Time: 14 minutes
Servings: 4
Ingredients:
- 2 lbs. rib eye steak, bone-in
- 1 tsp. fresh rosemary, chopped
- 1 tsp. fresh thyme, chopped
- 1 tsp. fresh chives, chopped
- 2 tsp. fresh parsley, chopped
- 1 tsp. garlic, minced
- ¼ cup butter softened
- Pepper to taste
- Salt to taste

Directions:
1. In a small bowl, combine butter and herbs.
2. Refrigerate the rib-eye steak for 30 minutes after rubbing it with herb butter.
3. Place the marinated steak on an Instant Vortex Air Fryer Oven pan and cook for 12–14 minutes at 400°F.
4. Serve and enjoy.

Nutrition:
- Calories: 416 Fat: 36.7 g.
- Carbohydrates 0.7 g. Protein: 20.3 g.

55. Honey Mustard Pork Tenderloin

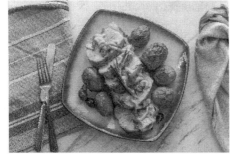

Preparation Time: 10 minutes
Cooking Time: 26 minutes
Servings: 4
Ingredients:
- 1 lb. pork tenderloin
- 1 tsp. sriracha sauce
- 1 tbsp. garlic, minced
- 2 tbsps. soy sauce
- 1 ½ tbsp. honey
- ¾ tbsp. Dijon mustard
- 1 tbsp. mustard

Directions:
1. Add sriracha sauce, garlic, soy sauce, honey, Dijon mustard, and mustard into the large zip-lock bag and mix well.
2. Add pork tenderloin into the bag. Seal bag and place in the fridge overnight. Preheat the Instant Vortex Air Fryer Oven to 380°F.
3. Spray Instant Vortex Air Fryer Tray with cooking spray then place marinated pork tenderloin on a tray and air fry for 26 minutes.
4. Turn pork tenderloin after every 5 minutes.
5. Slice and serve.

Nutrition:
- Calories: 195 Fat: 4.1 g.
- Carbohydrates 8 g. Protein: 30.5 g.

56. Simple Beef Sirloin Roast

Preparation Time: 10 minutes
Cooking Time: 50 minutes
Servings: 8
Ingredients:
- 2 ½ lbs. sirloin roast
- Salt and ground black pepper, as required

Directions:
1. Season the roast well with salt and black pepper.
2. Through the roast, insert the rotisserie rod.
3. To secure the rod to the bird, place one rotisserie fork on each side of the rod.
4. Place the drip pan in the cooking chamber of the Instant Vortex Plus Air Fryer Oven.
5. Select "Roast" and set the temperature to 350°F.
6. Press the "Start" button after setting the timer for 50 minutes.
7. Press the red lever down and load the left side of the rod into the Vortex when the display says "Add Food."
8. Now, slide the rod's left side into the metal bar's groove to keep it from moving. Then close the door and press the "Rotate" button. When the cooking time is up, press the red lever to release the rod.

9. Remove the roast from the Vortex and set it aside for 10 minutes before slicing. Cut the roast into desired-sized slices with a sharp knife and serve.

Nutrition:
- Calories: 201 Fat: 8.8 g.
- Carbohydrates 0 g.
- Protein: 28.9 g.

57. Seasoned Beef Roast

Preparation Time: 10 minutes
Cooking Time: 45 minutes
Servings: 10
Ingredients:
- 3 lbs. beef top roast
- 1 tbsp. olive oil
- 2 tbsps. Montreal steak seasoning

Directions:
1. Coat the roast with oil and then rub with the seasoning generously.
2. With kitchen twines, tie the roast to keep it compact. Arrange the roast onto the cooking tray.
3. Place the drip pan in the cooking chamber of the Instant Vortex Plus Air Fryer Oven.
4. Choose "Air Fry" and set the temperature to 360°F. Press the "Start" button after you set the timer for 45 minutes.
5. Place the cooking tray in the center position when the display says "Add Food."
6. Do nothing when the display says "Turn Food."
7. Remove the tray from the Vortex when the cooking time is up and set the roast on a platter for about 10 minutes before slicing. Cut the roast into desired-sized slices with a sharp knife and serve.

Nutrition:
- Calories: 259 Fat: 9.9 g.
- Carbohydrates 0 g.
- Fiber: 0 g.

58. Beef Burgers

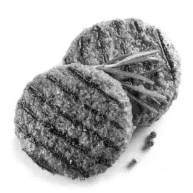

Preparation Time: 15 minutes
Cooking Time: 18 minutes
Servings: 4
Ingredients:
For the burgers:
- 1 lb. ground beef
- ½ cup panko breadcrumbs
- ¼ cup onion, chopped finely
- 3 tbsps. Dijon mustard
- 3 tsps. low-sodium soy sauce
- 2 tsps. fresh rosemary, chopped finely
- Salt, to taste

For the topping:
- 2 tbsps. Dijon mustard
- 1 tbsp. brown sugar
- 1 tsp. soy sauce
- 4 Gruyere cheese slices

Directions:
1. In a large bowl, add all ingredients and mix until well combined.
2. Make 4 equal-sized patties from the mixture.
3. Arrange the patties onto a cooking tray.
4. Arrange the drip pan in the bottom of the Instant Vortex Plus Air Fryer Oven cooking chamber.
5. Select "Air Fry" and then adjust the temperature to 370°F.
6. Set the timer for 15 minutes and press the "Start."
7. When the display shows "Add Food" insert the cooking rack in the center position.
8. When the display shows "Turn Food" turn the burgers.
9. Meanwhile, make the sauce by mixing the mustard, brown sugar, and soy sauce in a small basin.

10. Remove the tray from the Vortex after the cooking time is up and coat the burgers in the sauce.
11. 1 slice of cheese on top of each burger
12. Select "Broil" when returning the tray to the cooking chamber.
13. Press the "Start" button after setting the timer for 3 minutes.
14. Remove the dish from the Vortex after the cooking time is up and serve hot.

Nutrition:
- Calories: 412 Fat: 18 g.
- Carbohydrates 6.3 g. Protein: 44.4 g.

59. Season and Salt-Cured Beef

Preparation Time: 15 minutes
Cooking Time: 3 hours
Servings: 4
Ingredients:
- 1 ½ lb. beef round, trimmed
- ½ cup Worcestershire sauce
- ½ cup low-sodium soy sauce
- 2 tsps. honey
- 1 tsp. liquid smoke
- 2 tsps. onion powder
- ½ tsp. red pepper flakes
- Ground black pepper, as required

Directions:
1. In a bag zip-top, place the beef and freeze for 1–2 hours to firm up.
2. Place the meat onto a cutting board and cut against the grain into 1/8–¼-inch strips.
3. In a large bowl, add the remaining ingredients and mix until well combined.
4. Add the steak slices and coat with the mixture generously.
5. Refrigerate to marinate for about 4–6 hours.
6. Remove the beef slices from the bowl and with paper towels, pat dry them.
7. Arrange the steak pieces in an equal layer on the baking trays.
8. Choose "Dehydrate" and set the temperature to 160°F.
9. Press the "Start" button after setting the timer for 3 hours.
10. Insert one tray in the top position and the other in the center position when the display says "Add Food."
11. Switch the position of the cooking trays after 1–2 hours.
12. Meanwhile, boil the remaining ingredients in a small saucepan over medium heat for about 10 minutes, stirring regularly.
13. Remove the trays from the Vortex after the cooking time is finished.

Nutrition:
- Calories: 362 Fat: 10.7 g.
- Carbohydrates 11 g. Protein: 53.8 g.

60. Simple Beef Patties

Preparation Time: 10 minutes
Cooking Time: 13 minutes
Servings: 4
Ingredients:
- 1 lb. ground beef
- ½ tsp. garlic powder
- ¼ tsp. onion powder
- Pepper
- Salt

Directions:
1. Preheat the Instant Vortex Air Fryer Oven to 400°F.
2. Add ground meat, garlic powder, onion powder, pepper, and salt into the mixing bowl and mix until well combined.
3. Make even shape patties from the meat mixture and arrange them on the Air Fryer pan.
4. Place pan in instant vortex Air Fryer oven.
5. Cook patties for 10 minutes Turn patties after 5 minutes
6. Serve and enjoy.

Nutrition:
- Calories: 212 Fat: 7.1 g.
- Carbohydrates 0.4 g. Protein: 34.5 g.

61. Baked Tilapia Cheese

Preparation Time: 5-10 minutes
Cooking Time: 15 minutes
Servings: 1
Ingredients:
- 2 teaspoons Dijon mustard
- 1 teaspoon prepared horseradish
- 3 tablespoons mayonnaise
- 1 tablespoon lemon juice
- 1/4 cup dry bread crumbs
- 2 teaspoons butter, melted
- 2 tablespoons grated Parmesan cheese
- 2 tilapia fillets (5-6 ounces each)

Directions:
1. In a mixing bowl, add mayo, lemon juice, mustard, 1 tablespoon cheese, and horseradish. Combine to mix well with each other.

2. In another bowl, combine the remaining cheese, melted butter, and bread crumbs.
3. Place Instant Pot over kitchen platform. Place Air Fryer Lid on top. Press Air Fry, set the temperature to 375°F, and set the timer to 5 minutes to preheat. Press "Start" and allow it to preheat for 5 minutes.
4. Take Air Fryer Basket, grease it with some cooking spray. In the basket, add fish and top with the mayo mixture. Add the crumb mixture on top. Place the basket in the inner pot of Instant Pot, close the Air Fryer Lid on top. Press the "Bake" setting. Set temperature to 390°F and set the timer to 15 minutes. Press "Start."
5. Open Air Fryer Lid after cooking time is over. Serve warm.

Nutrition:
- Calories: 268 Fat: 7.5g
- Saturated Fat: 2g Trans Fat: 0g
- Carbohydrates: 8g Fiber: 0.5g
- Sodium: 624mg Protein: 28g

62. Breaded Cod Sticks

Preparation Time: 5 minutes
Cooking Time: 20 minutes
Servings: 1
Ingredients:
- 2 large eggs
- 3 tbsp. milk
- 2 cups breadcrumbs
- 1 cup almond flour
- 1 lb Cod

Directions:
1. Heat the Air Fryer at 350° Fahrenheit.
2. Prepare three bowls one with the milk and eggs, one with the breadcrumbs (salt and pepper if desired), and another with almond flour.
3. Dip the sticks in the flour, egg mixture, and breadcrumbs.
4. Place in the basket and set the timer for 12 minutes. Toss the basket halfway through the cooking process.
5. Serve with your favorite sauce.

Nutrition:
- Calories 254
- Fat 14.2 g
- Carbohydrates 5.7 g
- Protein 39.1 g

63. Shrimp, Zucchini and Cherry Tomato Sauce

Preparation Time: 5 minutes
Cooking Time: 30 minutes
Servings: 1
Ingredients:
- 2 zucchinis
- 300 shrimp
- 7 cherry tomatoes
- Salt and pepper to taste
- 1 clove garlic

Directions:
1. Pour the oil into the Air Fryer, add the garlic clove, and diced zucchini.
2. Cook for 15 minutes at 150°C
3. Add the shrimp and the pieces of tomato, salt, and spices.
4. Cook for another 5 to 10 minutes or until the shrimp water evaporates.

Nutrition:
- Calories: 214.3 Fat: 8.6g
- Carbohydrates: 7.8g Sugar: 4.8g
- Protein: 27.0g Cholesterol: 232.7mg

64. Honey Glazed Salmon

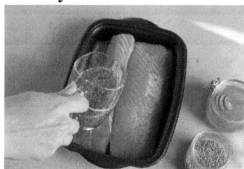

Preparation Time: 10 minutes
Cooking Time: 8 minutes
Servings: 1
Ingredients:
- 2 (6-oz.) salmon fillets
- Salt, as required
- 2 tablespoons honey

Directions:
1. Sprinkle the salmon fillets with salt and then, coat with honey.
2. Press "Power Button" of Air Fry Oven and turn the dial to select the "Air Fry" mode.
3. Press the Time button and again turn the dial to set the Cooking Time to 8 minutes.
4. Now push the Temp button and rotate the dial to set the temperature at 355 degrees F.

5. Press "Start/Pause" button to start.
6. When the unit beeps to show that it is preheated, open the lid.
7. Arrange the salmon fillets in greased "Air Fry Basket" and insert in the oven.
8. Serve hot.

Nutrition:
- Calories: 289
- Fat: 10.5 g
- Carbohydrates: 17.3 g
- Protein: 33.1 g

65. Crumbled Fish

Preparation Time: 5 minutes
Cooking Time: 15 minutes
Servings: 1
Ingredients:
- ½ cup breadcrumbs
- 4 tbsp. vegetable oil
- 1 egg
- 4 Fish fillets
- 1 Lemon

Directions:
1. Heat the Air Fryer to reach 356° Fahrenheit.
2. Whisk the oil and breadcrumbs until crumbly.
3. Dip the fish into the egg, then the crumb mixture.
4. Arrange the fish in the cooker and Air fry for 12 minutes.
5. Garnish using the lemon.

Nutrition:
- Calories: 320 Carbohydrates: 8 g
- Fat: 10 g Protein: 28 g

66. Salted Marinated Salmon

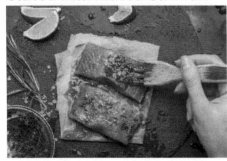

Preparation Time: 10 minutes
Cooking Time: 30 minutes
Servings: 1
Ingredients:
- 500 g salmon fillet
- 1 kg coarse salt

Directions:
1. Place the baking paper on the Air Fryer basket and the salmon on top (skin side up) covered with coarse salt.
2. Set the Air Fryer to 150°C
3. Cook everything for 25 to 30 minutes. At the end of cooking, remove the salt from the fish and serve with a drizzle of oil.

Nutrition:
- Calories: 290
- Fat: 13g
- Carbohydrates: 3g
- Fiber: 0g
- Protein: 40g
- Cholesterol: 196mg

67. Sautéed Trout with Almonds

Preparation Time: 35 minutes
Cooking Time: 20 minutes
Servings: 1
Ingredients:
- 700 g salmon trout
- 15 black peppercorns
- Dill leaves to taste
- 30g almonds
- Salt to taste

Directions:
1. Cut the trout into cubes and marinate it for half an hour with the rest of the ingredients (except salt).
2. Cook in the Air Fryer for 17 minutes at 1600CUP Pour a drizzle of oil and serve.

Nutrition:
- Calories: 238.5
- Fat: 20.1 g
- Carbohydrates: 11.5 g
- Sugar: 1.0 g
- Protein: 4.0 g
- Cholesterol: 45.9 mg

68. Cod Fish Nuggets

Preparation Time: 5 minutes
Cooking Time: 20 minutes
Servings: 1
Ingredients:
- 1 lb Cod fillet
- 3 eggs
- 4 tbsp. olive oil
- 1 cup almond flour
- 1 cup Gluten-free breadcrumbs

Directions:
1. Heat the Air Fryer at 390° Fahrenheit.
2. Slice the cod into nuggets.
3. Prepare three bowls. Whisk the eggs in one. Combine the salt, oil, and breadcrumbs in another. Sift the almond flour into the third one.
4. Cover each of the nuggets with flour, dip in the eggs, and the breadcrumbs.
5. Arrange the nuggets in the basket and set the timer for 20 minutes.
6. Serve the fish with your favorite dips or sides.

Nutrition:
- Calories: 334
- Fat: 10g
- Carbohydrates: 8 g
- Protein: 32g

69. Creamy Salmon

Preparation Time: 5 minutes
Cooking Time: 20 minutes
Servings: 1
Ingredients:
- 1 tbsp. chopped dill
- 1 tbsp. olive oil
- 3 tbsp. sour cream
- 1.76 oz. plain yogurt
- 6 pieces/0.75 lb. salmon

Directions:
1. Heat the Air Fryer and wait for it to reach 285° Fahrenheit.
2. Shake the salt over the salmon and add them to the fryer basket with the olive oil to Air fry for 10 minutes.
3. Whisk the yogurt, salt, and dill.
4. Serve the salmon with the sauce with your favorite sides.

Nutrition:
- Calories: 340
- Carbohydrates: 5 g
- Fat: 16 g
- Protein: 32 g

70. Baked Onion Cod

Preparation Time: 10 minutes
Cooking Time: 12 minutes
Servings: 1
Ingredients:
- 1/2 pound thick-cut cod loin
- 1/4 lemon juice
- 2 tablespoons butter, melted
- 1/4 sleeve round crackers, crushed
- 1 1/2 teaspoons chopped parsley
- 1 1/2 teaspoons chopped green onion
- 1/2 lemon, cut into wedges
- 2 tablespoons dry white wine

Directions:
1. In a mixing bowl, add half butter and crackers. Combine to mix well with each other.
2. In another bowl, add lemon juice, white wine, parsley, and green onion. Combine to mix well with each other. Coat cod with remaining butter.
3. Place Instant Pot over kitchen platform. Place Air Fryer Lid on top. Press Air Fry, set the temperature to 375°F, and set the timer to 5 minutes to preheat. Press "Start" and allow it to preheat for 5 minutes.
4. Take Air Fryer Basket, grease it with some cooking spray. In the basket, add cod. Top with the dressing and add the cracker mixture on top.
5. Place the basket in the inner pot of Instant Pot, close the Air Fryer Lid on top. Press the "Bake" setting. Set temperature to 390°F and set the timer to 10 minutes. Press "Start."
6. Open Air Fryer Lid after cooking time is over. Serve warm.

Nutrition:
- Calories: 290 Fat: 15g
- Saturated Fat: 3g
- Trans Fat: 0g
- Carbohydrates: 10g
- Fiber: 2g
- Sodium: 624mg
- Protein: 21g

71. Mussels with Pepper

Preparation Time: 15 minutes
Cooking Time: 20 minutes
Servings: 1
Ingredients:
- 700g mussels
- 1 clove garlic
- 1 tsp oil
- Pepper to taste
- Parsley Taste

Directions:
1. Clean and scrape the mold cover and remove the byssus (the "beard" that comes out of the mold).

2. Pour the oil, clean the mussels and the crushed garlic in the Air Fryer basket. Set the temperature to 2000C and simmer for 12 minutes. Towards the end of cooking, add black pepper and chopped parsley.
3. Finally, distribute the mussel juice well at the bottom of the basket, stirring the basket.

Nutrition:
- Calories: 150
- Carbohydrates: 2g
- Fat: 8g
- Sugar: 0g
- Protein: 15g
- Cholesterol: 0mg

72. Cajun Salmon

Preparation Time: 5 minutes
Cooking Time: 10 minutes
Servings: 1
Ingredients:
- 1 - 7 oz. / 0.75-inches thick salmon fillet
- Cajun seasoning
- ¼ lemon juice
- Optional: Sprinkle of sugar

Directions:
1. Set the Air Fryer at 356° Fahrenheit to preheat for five minutes.
2. Rinse and dry the salmon with a paper towel. Cover the fish with the Cajun coating mix.
3. Place the fillet in the Air Fryer for seven minutes with the skin side up.
4. Serve with a sprinkle of lemon and dusting of sugar if desired.

Nutrition:
- Calories: 285
- Fat: 17.8 g
- Carbohydrates: 6.8 g
- Protein: 42.1 g

73. Breaded Flounder

Preparation Time: 15 minutes
Cooking Time: 12 minutes
Servings: 1
Ingredients:
- 1 egg
- 1 cup dry breadcrumbs
- ¼ cup vegetable oil
- 3 (6-oz.) flounder fillets
- 1 lemon, sliced

Directions:
1. In a shallow bowl, beat the egg
2. In another bowl, add the breadcrumbs and oil and mix until a crumbly mixture is formed.
3. Dip flounder fillets into the beaten egg and then, coat with the breadcrumb mixture.
4. Press "Power Button" of Air Fry Oven and turn the dial to select the "Air Fry" mode.
5. Press the Time button and again turn the dial to set the Cooking Time to 12 minutes.
6. Now push the Temp button and rotate the dial to set the temperature at 356 degrees F.
7. Press "Start/Pause" button to start.
8. When the unit beeps to show that it is preheated, open the lid.
9. Arrange the flounder fillets in greased "Air Fry Basket" and insert it in the oven.
10. Plate with lemon slices and serve hot.

Nutrition:
- Calories: 524
- Total Fat: 24.2 g
- Saturated Fat: 5.1 g
- Cholesterol: 170 mg
- Sodium: 463 mg
- Total Carbs: 26.5 g
- Fiber: 1.5 g
- Sugar: 2.5 g
- Protein: 47.8g

74. Caramelized Salmon Fillet

Preparation Time: 5 minutes
Cooking Time: 25 minutes
Servings: 1
Ingredients:
- 2 salmon fillets
- 60g cane sugar
- 4 tbsp soy sauce
- 50g sesame seeds
- Unlimited Ginger

Directions:
1. Preheat the Air Fryer at 180°C for 5 minutes.
2. Put the sugar and soy sauce in the basket.
3. Cook everything for 5 minutes.
4. In the meantime, wash the fish well, pass it through sesame to cover it completely and place it inside the tank and add the fresh ginger.
5. Cook for 12 minutes.

6. Turn the fish over and finish cooking for another 8 minutes.

Nutrition:
- Calories: 569
- Fat: 14.9 g
- Carbohydrates: 40 g
- Sugar: 27.6 g
- Protein: 66.9 g
- Cholesterol: 165.3 mg

75. Salmon Butter Crumbed

Preparation Time: 5-10 minutes
Cooking Time: 10 minutes
Servings: 1
Ingredients:
- 1 tablespoon thyme, chopped
- 2 garlic cloves, minced
- 1 1/2 cups soft bread crumbs
- 2 tablespoons minced parsley
- 1 teaspoon grated lemon zest
- 1/2 teaspoon salt
- 1/4 teaspoon paprika
- 1 tablespoon butter, melted
- 1/4 teaspoon lemon-pepper seasoning
- 2 salmon fillets (6 ounces each)

Directions:
1. In a mixing bowl, add bread crumbs, fresh parsley thyme, garlic, lemon zest, salt, lemon-pepper seasoning, and paprika. Combine to mix well with each other.
2. Place Instant Pot over kitchen platform. Place Air Fryer Lid on top. Press Air Fry, set the temperature to 375°F, and set the timer to 5 minutes to preheat. Press "Start" and allow it to preheat for 5 minutes.
3. Take Air Fryer Basket, grease it with some cooking spray. In the basket, add salmon fillets skin side down and top with the crumb mixture.
4. Place the basket in the inner pot of Instant Pot, close Air Fryer Lid on top.
5. Press the "Bake" setting. Set temperature to 390°F and set the timer to 10 minutes. Press "Start."
6. Open Air Fryer Lid after cooking time is over. Serve warm.

Nutrition:
- Calories: 308 Fat: 17g
- Saturated Fat: 2.5g Trans Fat: 0g
- Carbohydrates: 11.5g Fiber: 1g
- Sodium: 347mg
- Protein: 9g

76. Cajun Shrimp

Preparation Time: 5 minutes
Cooking Time: 5 minutes
Servings: 1
Ingredients:
- 16-20/1.25 lb. Tiger shrimp
- 1 tbsp. olive oil
- ½ tsp. Old Bay seasoning
- ½ tsp. smoked paprika
- ½ tsp. cayenne pepper

Directions:
1. Set the Air Fryer at 390° Fahrenheit.
2. Cover the shrimp using the oil and spices.
3. Toss them into the Air Fryer basket and set the timer for five minutes.
4. Serve with your favorite side dish.

Nutrition:
- Calories: 356
- Fat: 18g
- Carbohydrates: 5 g
- Protein: 34g

77. Vegetable Egg Halibut

Preparation Time: 5-10 minutes
Cooking Time: 15 miutes
Servings: 1-6
Ingredients:
- 2 pounds mixed vegetables
- 4 cups torn lettuce leaves
- 1 cup cherry tomatoes, halved
- 1 ½ pound halibut fillets
- Black pepper (ground) and salt to taste
- 2 tablespoons olive oil
- 4 large hard-boiled eggs, sliced

Directions:
1. Rub the halibut with salt and black pepper. Coat fish with oil.
2. Place Instant Pot over kitchen platform. Place Air Fryer Lid on top. Press Air Fry, set the temperature to 375°F, and set the timer to 5 minutes to preheat. Press "Start" and allow it to preheat for 5 minutes.
3. Take Air Fryer Basket, grease it with some cooking spray. In the basket, add fish and arrange vegetables around.
4. Place the basket in the inner pot of Instant Pot, close Air Fryer Lid on top.
5. Press the "Air Fry" setting. Set temperature to 375°F and set the timer to 15 minutes. Press "Start." Stir the mixture halfway down.

6. Open Air Fryer Lid after cooking time is over. Serve warm in a bowl mixed with eggs, lettuce, and tomatoes.

Nutrition:
- Calories: 336
- Fat: 11g
- Saturated Fat: 3g
- Trans Fat: 0g
- Carbohydrates: 16g
- Fiber: 2g
- Sodium: 658mg
- Protein: 20.5g

78. Deep Fried Prawns

Preparation Time: 15 minutes
Cooking Time: 20 minutes
Servings: 1
Ingredients:
- 12 prawns
- 2 eggs
- Flour to taste
- Breadcrumbs
- 1 tsp. oil

Directions:
- Remove the head of the prawns and shell carefully.
- Pass the prawns first in the flour, then in the beaten egg, and then in the breadcrumbs.
- Preheat the Air Fryer for 1 minute at 150°C
- Add the prawns and cook for 4 minutes. If the prawns are large, it will be necessary to cook 6 at a time.
- Turn the prawns and cook for another 4 minutes.
- They should be served with a yogurt or mayonnaise sauce.

Nutrition:
- Calorie0:s 2385.1
- Fat: 23 g
- Carbohydrates: 52.3g
- Sugar: 0.1g
- Protein: 21.4g

CHAPTER 9:

Recipes for Dinner

79. Brine-Soaked Turkey

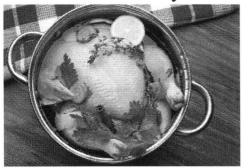

Preparation Time: 10 minutes
Cooking Time: 45 minutes
Servings: 8
Ingredients:

- 7 lb. bone-in, skin-on turkey breast

For the brine:

- ½ cup salt
- 1 lemon
- ½ onion
- 3 cloves garlic, smashed
- 5 sprigs of fresh thyme
- 3 bay leaves - Black pepper

For the turkey breast:

- 4 tbsps. butter, softened
- ½ tsp. black pepper
- ½ tsp. garlic powder
- ¼ tsp. dried thyme
- ¼ tsp. dried oregano

Directions:

1. Mix the turkey brine ingredients in a pot and soak the turkey in the brine overnight. The next day, remove the soaked turkey from the brine.
2. Whisk the butter, black pepper, garlic powder, oregano, and thyme. Brush the butter mixture over the turkey then places it in a baking tray.
3. To select the "Air Roast" mode, press the "Power Button" on the Air Fry Oven and spin the dial. To set the cooking time to 45 minutes, press the "Time" button and then turn the dial again.
4. To set the temperature, press the "Temp" button and rotate the dial to 370°F. Place the turkey baking pan in the oven and close the cover once it has been preheated.
5. Slice and serve warm.

Nutrition:

- Calories: 397 Fat: 15.4 g.
- Carbohydrates 58.5 g.
- Protein: 7.9 g.

80. Oregano Chicken Breast

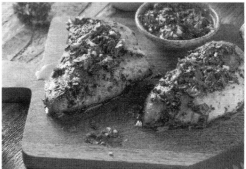

Preparation Time: 10 minutes
Cooking Time: 25 minutes
Servings: 6
Ingredients:

- 2 lbs. chicken breasts, minced
- 1 tbsp. avocado oil
- 1 tsp. smoked paprika
- 1 tsp. garlic powder
- 1 tsp. oregano
- ½ tsp. salt
- Black pepper, to taste

Directions:

1. Toss all the meatball ingredients in a bowl and mix well. Make small meatballs out of this mixture and place them in the Air Fryer basket.
2. Press the "Power Button" of Air Fry Oven and turn the dial to select the "Air Fry" mode. Press the "Time" button and again turn the dial to set the cooking time to 25 minutes
3. Now push the "Temp" button and rotate the dial to set the temperature at 375°F.

4. Once preheated, place the Air Fryer basket inside and close its lid.
5. Serve warm.

Nutrition:
- Calories: 352
- Fat: 14 g
- Carbohydrates: 15.8 g
- Protein: 26 g

81. Thyme Turkey Breast

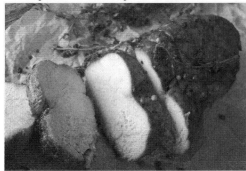

Preparation Time: 10 minutes
Cooking Time: 40 minutes
Servings: 4
Ingredients:
- 2 lbs. turkey breast
- Salt, to taste
- Black pepper, to taste
- 4 tbsps. butter, melted
- 3 cloves garlic, minced
- 1 tsp. thyme, chopped
- 1 tsp. rosemary, chopped

Directions:
1. Mix butter with salt, black pepper, garlic, thyme, and rosemary in a bowl.
2. Rub this seasoning over the turkey breast liberally and place it in the Air Fryer basket.
3. Turn the dial to select the "Air Fry" mode.
4. Hit the "Time" button and again use the dial to set the cooking time to 40 minutes.
5. Now push the "Temp" button and rotate the dial to set the temperature at 375°F.
6. Once preheated, place the Air Fryer basket inside the oven.
7. Slice and serve fresh.

Nutrition:
- Calories: 334
- Fat: 4.7 g.
- Carbohydrates 54.1 g.
- Protein: 26.2 g.

82. Chicken Drumsticks

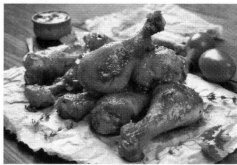

Preparation Time: 10 minutes
Cooking Time: 20 minutes
Servings: 8
Ingredients:
- 8 chicken drumsticks
- 2 tbsps. olive oil
- 1 tsp. salt
- 1 tsp. pepper
- 1 tsp. garlic powder
- 1 tsp. paprika
- ½ tsp. cumin

Directions:
1. Mix olive oil with salt, black pepper, garlic powder, paprika, and cumin in a bowl.
2. Rub this mixture liberally over all the drumsticks.
3. Place these drumsticks in the Air Fryer basket.
4. Turn the dial to select the "Air Fry" mode.
5. Hit the "Time" button and again use the dial to set the cooking time to 20 minutes.
6. Now push the "Temp" button and rotate the dial to set the temperature at 375°F.
7. Once preheated, place the Air Fryer basket inside the oven.
8. Flip the drumsticks when cooked halfway through.
9. Resume air frying for another rest of the 10 minutes.
10. Serve warm.

Nutrition:
- Calories: 212
- Fat: 11.8 g.
- Carbohydrates: 14.6 g.
- Protein: 17.3 g.

83. Lemon Chicken Breasts

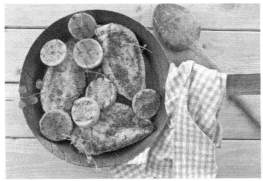

Preparation Time: 10 minutes
Cooking Time: 30 minutes
Servings: 4
Ingredients:

- 1/3 cup white wine, dry
- 4 boneless skin-on chicken breasts
- 1 sliced lemon
- 1 tbsp. grated lemon zest
- 2 tbsps. lemon juice
- 1 ½ tbsp. crushed dried oregano
- 1 tsp. chopped thyme leaves
- black pepper and salt to taste
- ¼ cup extra virgin olive oil
- 3 tsps. minced garlic

Directions:
1. In a baking pan, whisk together all ingredients to thoroughly coat the chicken breasts.
2. Serve the chicken breasts with lemon wedges on top.
3. Over the toasted bread slices, spread the mustard mixture.
4. To select the "Bake" mode, press the "Power Button" on the Air Fry Oven and spin the dial.
5. To set the cooking time to 30 minutes, press the "Time" button and then turn the dial again.
6. To set the temperature, press the "Temp" button and rotate the dial to 370°F.
7. Place the baking pan inside and close the lid once the oven has been warmed.
8. Warm the dish before serving.

Nutrition:
- Calories: 388
- Fat: 8 g.
- Carbohydrates: 8 g.
- Protein: 13 g.

84. Parmesan Chicken Meatballs

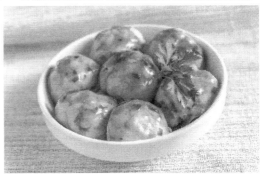

Preparation Time: 10 minutes
Cooking Time: 12 minutes
Servings: 4
Ingredients:

- 1 lb. ground chicken
- 1 large egg, beaten
- ½ cup Parmesan cheese, grated
- ½ cup pork rinds, ground
- 1 tsp. garlic powder
- 1 tsp. paprika
- 1 tsp. kosher salt
- ½ tsp. pepper

For the crust:

- ½ cup pork rinds, ground

Directions:
1. Toss all the meatball ingredients in a bowl and mix well. Make small meatballs out of this mixture and roll them in the pork rinds.
2. Place the coated meatballs in the Air Fryer basket. Select "Power Button" of Air Fry Oven and turn the control to select the "Bake" mode.
3. Press the "Time" button and again turn the control to set the cooking time to 12 minutes. Now push the "Temp" button and rotate the dial to set the temperature at 400°F.
4. Once preheated, place the Air Fryer basket inside and close its lid.
5. Serve warm.

Nutrition:
- Calories: 529
- Fat: 17 g.
- Carbohydrates: 55 g.
- Protein: 41 g.

85. Easy Italian Meatballs

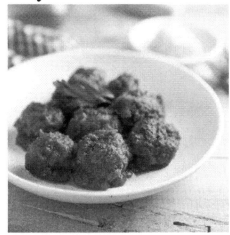

Preparation Time: 10 minutes
Cooking Time: 13 minutes
Servings: 4
Ingredients:

- 2 lbs. lean ground turkey
- ¼ cup onion, minced
- 2 cloves garlic, minced
- 2 tbsps. parsley, chopped
- 2 eggs
- 1 ½ cup parmesan cheese, grated
- ½ tsp. red pepper flakes
- ½ tsp. Italian seasoning
- Salt and black pepper to taste

Directions:

1. Toss all the meatball ingredients in a bowl and mix well. Make small meatballs out of this mixture and place them in the Air Fryer basket.
2. Select the "Air Fry" mode by pressing the "Power Button" on the Air Fry Oven and turning the dial. To set the cooking time to 13 minutes, press the "Time" button and then turn the dial again. To set the temperature, press the "Temp" button and crank the dial to 350°F.
3. Once preheated, place the Air Fryer basket inside and close its lid.
4. Flip the meatballs when cooked halfway through.
5. Serve warm.

Nutrition:

- Calories: 472
- Fat: 25.8
- Carbohydrates: 1.7 g.
- Protein: 59.6 g.

86. Buttered Salmon

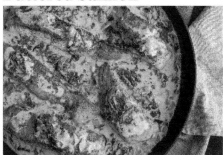

Preparation Time: 5 minutes
Cooking Time: 10 minutes
Servings: 2
Ingredients:

- 2 (6 oz.) salmon fillets
- Salt and ground black pepper, as required
- 1 tbsp. butter, melted

Directions:

1. Season each salmon fillet with salt and black pepper and then, coat with the butter. Arrange the salmon fillets onto the greased cooking tray.
2. Arrange the drip pan in the bottom of the Instant Vortex Air Fryer Oven cooking chamber. Select "Air Fry" and then adjust the temperature to 360°F. Set the time for 10 minutes and press "Start."
3. When the display shows "Add Food" insert the cooking tray in the center position. When the display shows "Turn Food" turn the salmon fillets.
4. When cooking time is complete, remove the tray from the Vortex Oven. Serve hot.

Nutrition:

- Calories: 276 Carbohydrates: 0 g.
- Fat: 16.3 g. Protein: 33.1 g.

87. Crispy Haddock

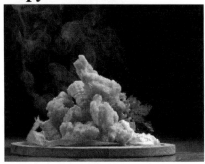

Preparation Time: 5 minutes
Cooking Time: 10 minutes
Servings: 3
Ingredients:

- ½ cup flour

- ½ tsp. paprika
- 1 egg, beaten
- ¼ cup mayonnaise
- 4 oz. salt and vinegar potato chips, crushed finely
- 1 lb. haddock fillet cut into 6 pieces

Directions:
1. In a shallow dish, mix the flour and paprika. In a second shallow dish, add the egg and mayonnaise and beat well. In a third shallow dish, place the crushed potato chips.
2. Coat the fish pieces with flour mixture, then dip into the egg mixture, and finally coat with the potato chips. Arrange the fish pieces onto 2 cooking trays.
3. Place the drip pan in the cooking chamber of the Instant Vortex Air Fryer Oven. Select "Air Fry" and set the temperature to 370°F. Set the timer for 10 minutes and hit the "Start" button.
4. Insert one cooking tray in the top position and another in the bottom position when the display says "Add Food."
5. When the display says "Turn Food," don't turn the food instead, move the cooking trays around. Remove the trays from the Vortex Oven when the cooking time is up. Serve immediately.

Nutrition:
- Calories: 456
- Carbohydrates: 40.9 g.
- Fat: 22.7 g.
- Protein: 43.5 g.

88. Miso Glazed Salmon

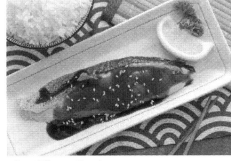

Preparation Time: 5 minutes
Cooking Time: 10 minutes
Servings: 4
Ingredients:
- 1/3 cups sake
- ¼ cups sugar
- ¼ cups red miso
- 1 tbsp. low-sodium soy sauce
- 2 tbsps. vegetable oil
- 4 (5 oz.) skinless salmon fillets, 1-inch thick

Directions:
1. Place's sake, sugar, miso, soy sauce, and oil into a bowl and beat until thoroughly combined. Rub the salmon fillets with the mixture generously. In a plastic zip-lock bag, place the salmon fillets with any remaining miso mixture.
2. Seal the bag and refrigerate to marinate for about 30 minutes Grease a baking dish that will fit in the Vortex Air Fryer Oven. Remove the salmon fillets from the bag and shake off the excess marinade. Arrange the salmon fillets into the prepared baking dish.
3. Place the drip pan in the bottom of the Instant Vortex Air Fryer Oven cooking chamber. Select "Broil" and set the time for 5 minutes.
4. When the display shows "Add Food" insert the baking dish in the center position.
5. When the display shows "Turn Food" do not turn the food. When cooking time is complete, remove the baking dish from the Vortex Oven. Serve hot.

Nutrition:
- Calories: 335 Carbohydrates: 18.3 g.
- Fat: 16.6 g.
- Protein: 29.8 g.

89. Ground Chicken Meatballs

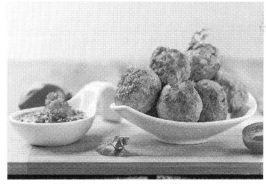

Preparation Time: 10 minutes
Cooking Time: 10 minutes
Servings: 4
Ingredients:
- 1 lb. ground chicken
- 1/3 cup panko
- 1 tsp. salt
- 2 tsps. chives
- ½ tsp. garlic powder
- 1 tsp. thyme
- 1 egg

Directions:
1. Toss all the meatball ingredients in a bowl and mix well. Make small meatballs out of this mixture and place them in the Air Fryer basket.
2. Press the "Power Button" of Air Fry Oven and turn the dial to select the "Air Fry" mode. Press the "Time" button and again turn the dial to set the cooking time to 10 minutes.
3. Now push the "Temp" button and rotate the dial to set the temperature at 350°F. Once preheated, place the Air Fryer basket inside and close its lid. Serve warm.

Nutrition:
- Calories: 453 Fat: 2.4 g.
- Carbohydrates: 18 g.
- Protein: 23.2 g.

90. Lemony Salmon

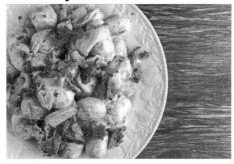

Preparation Time: 5 minutes
Cooking Time: 10 minutes
Servings: 2
Ingredients:
- 1 tbsp. fresh lemon juice
- ½ tbsp. olive oil
- Salt and ground black pepper, as required
- 1 garlic clove, minced
- ½ tsp. fresh thyme leaves, chopped
- 2 (7 oz.) salmon fillets

Directions:
1. Combine all ingredients in a mixing dish, except the salmon, and stir thoroughly. Add the salmon fillets and generously cover them in the mixture.
2. Place the salmon fillets skin-side down on a lightly greased frying rack. Place the drip pan in the cooking chamber of the Instant Vortex Air Fryer Oven. Select "Air Fry" and set the temperature to 400°F. Set the timer for 10 minutes and hit the "Start" button.
3. Place the frying rack in the bottom position when the display says "Add Food." Turn the fillets when the display says "Turn Food."
4. Remove the tray from the Vortex Oven after the cooking time is over. Serve immediately.

Nutrition:
- Calories: 297
- Carbohydrates: 0.8 g.
- Fat: 15.8 g.
- Protein: 38.7 g.

91. Crispy Tilapia

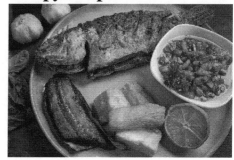

Preparation Time: 5 minutes
Cooking Time: 15 minutes
Servings: 2
Ingredients:
- ¾ cup cornflakes, crushed
- 1 (1 oz.) packet dry ranch-style dressing mix
- 2 ½ tbsps. vegetable oil
- 2 eggs
- 4 (6 oz.) tilapia fillets

Directions:
1. In a shallow bowl, beat the eggs. In another bowl, add the cornflakes, ranch dressing, and oil and mix until a crumbly mixture forms. Dip the fish fillets into the egg and then, coat with the cornflake mixture.
2. Arrange the tilapia fillets onto the greased cooking tray. Arrange the drip pan in the bottom of the Instant Vortex Air Fryer Oven cooking chamber. Select "Air Fry" and then adjust the temperature to 355°F. Set the time for 14 minutes and press "Start."
3. When the display shows "Add Food" insert the cooking tray in the center position. When the display shows "Turn Food" turn the tilapia fillets. When cooking time is complete, remove the tray from the Vortex Oven.
4. Serve hot.

Nutrition:
- Calories: 291 Carbohydrates: 4.9 g.
- Fat: 14.6 g. Protein: 34.8 g.

92. Vinegar Halibut

Preparation Time: 5 minutes
Cooking Time: 12 minutes
Servings: 2
Ingredients:

- 2 (5 oz.) halibut fillets
- 1 garlic clove, minced
- 1 tsp. fresh rosemary, minced
- 1 tbsp. olive oil
- 1 tbsp. red wine vinegar
- 1/8 tsp. hot sauce

Directions:

1. In a large resealable bag, add all ingredients. Seal the bag and shale well to mix. Refrigerate to marinate for at least 30 minutes. Remove the fish fillets from the bag and shake off the excess marinade. Arrange the halibut fillets onto the greased cooking tray.
2. Place the drip pan in the cooking chamber of the Instant Vortex Air Fryer Oven. Select "Bake" and set the temperature to 450°F. Set the timer for 12 minutes and hit the "Start" button. Place the cooking tray in the center position when the display says "Add Food." Turn the halibut fillets when the display says "Turn Food." Remove the tray from the Vortex Oven after the cooking time is over. Serve immediately.

Nutrition:

- Calories: 223 Carbohydrates: 1 g.
- Fat: 10.4 g.
- Protein: 30 g.

93. Crusted Chicken Drumsticks

Preparation Time: 10 minutes
Cooking Time: 10 minutes
Servings: 4
Ingredients:

- 1 lb. chicken drumsticks
- ½ cup buttermilk
- ½ cup panko breadcrumbs
- ½ cup flour
- ¼ tsp. baking powder

For the spice mixture:

- ½ tsp. salt
- ½ tsp. celery salt
- ¼ tsp. oregano
- ¼ tsp. cayenne - 1 tsp. paprika
- ¼ tsp. garlic powder
- ¼ tsp. dried thyme
- ½ tsp. ground ginger
- ½ tsp. white pepper
- ½ tsp. black pepper
- 3 tbsps. butter melted

Directions:

1. Soak chicken in the buttermilk and cover to marinate overnight in the refrigerator. Mix spices with flour, breadcrumbs, and baking powder in a shallow tray.
2. Remove the chicken from the milk and coat them well with the flour spice mixture.
3. Place the chicken drumsticks in the Air Fryer basket of the Ninja Oven.
4. Pour the melted butter over the drumsticks.
5. Turn the dial to select the "Air Fry" mode. Hit the "Time" button and again use the dial to set the cooking time to 10 minutes.
6. Now push the "Temp" button and rotate the dial to set the temperature at 425°F.
7. Once preheated, place the baking tray inside the oven.
8. Flip the drumsticks and resume cooking for another 10 minutes.
9. 9 Serve warm.

Nutrition:

- Calories: 331 Fat: 2.5 g.
- Carbohydrates: 69 g. Protein: 28.7 g.

94. Spiced Tilapia

Preparation Time: 5 minutes
Cooking Time: 12 minutes
Servings: 2
Ingredients:

- ½ tsp. lemon-pepper seasoning
- ½ tsp. garlic powder
- ½ tsp. onion powder
- Salt and ground black pepper, as required
- 2 (6 oz.) tilapia fillets
- 1 tbsp. olive oil

Directions:

1. In a small bowl, mix the spices, salt, and black pepper. Coat the tilapia fillets with oil and then rub with spice mixture. Arrange the tilapia fillets onto a lightly greased cooking rack, skin-side down.
2. Arrange the drip pan in the bottom of the Instant Vortex Air Fryer Oven cooking chamber. Select "Air Fry" and then adjust the temperature to 360°F. Set the time for 12 minutes and press "Start."

3. Place the frying rack in the lowest position when the display says "Add Food." Turn the fillets when the display says "Turn Food."
4. When the time of cooking is complete, remove the tray from the Vortex Oven. Serve hot.

Nutrition:
- Calories: 206
- Carbohydrates: 0.2 g. Fat: 8.6 g.
- Protein: 31.9 g.

95. Simple Haddock

Preparation Time: 5 minutes
Cooking Time: 10 minutes
Servings: 2
Ingredients:
- 2 (6 oz.) haddock fillets
- 1 tbsp. olive oil
- Salt and ground black pepper, as required

Directions:
1. Coat the haddock fillets with oil and then, sprinkle with salt and black pepper. Arrange the haddock fillets onto a greased cooking rack and spray with cooking spray.
2. Place the drip pan in the bottom of the Instant Vortex Air Fryer Oven cooking chamber. Select "Air Fry" and then adjust the temperature to 355°F. Set the time for 8 minutes and press "Start."
3. When the display shows "Add Food" insert the cooking rack in the center position.
4. When the display shows "Turn Food" do not turn the food.
5. When the cooking time is complete, remove the rack from the Vortex Oven. Serve hot.

Nutrition:
- Calories: 251 Carbohydrates: 0 g.
- Fat: 8.6 g.
- Protein: 41.2 g.

96. Breaded Cod

Preparation Time: 5 minutes
Cooking Time: 10 minutes
Servings: 4
Ingredients:
- 1/3 cup all-purpose flour
- Ground black pepper, as required
- 1 large egg
- 2 tbsps. water
- 2/3 cup cornflakes, crushed
- 1 tbsp. parmesan cheese, grated
- 1/8 tsp. cayenne pepper
- 1 lb. cod fillets
- Salt, as required

Directions:
1. In a shallow dish, add the flour and black pepper and mix well. In a second shallow dish, add the egg and water and beat well. In a third shallow dish, add the cornflakes, cheese, and cayenne pepper and mix well.
2. Season the cod fillets with salt evenly. Coat the fillets with flour mixture, then dip into the egg mixture and finally coat with the cornflake mixture. Arrange the cod fillets onto the greased cooking rack. Arrange the drip pan in the bottom of the Instant Vortex Air Fryer Oven cooking chamber. Select "Air Fry" and then adjust the temperature to 400°F. Set the time for 15 minutes and press "Start."
3. Place the frying rack in the lowest position when the display says "Add Food." Turn the fish fillets when the display says "Turn Food." Remove the tray from the Vortex Oven after the cooking time is over. Serve immediately.

Nutrition:
- Calories: 168 Carbohydrates: 12.1 g.
- Fat: 2.7 g. Protein: 23.7 g.

97. Spicy Catfish

Preparation Time: 5 minutes
Cooking Time: 15 minutes
Servings: 4
Ingredients:
- 2 tbsps. cornmeal polenta
- 2 tsp. Cajun seasoning
- ½ tsp. paprika
- ½ tsp. garlic powder
- Salt, as required
- 2 (6 oz.) catfish fillets
- 1 tbsp. olive oil

Directions:
1. In a bowl, mix cornmeal, Cajun seasoning, paprika, garlic powder, and salt. Add catfish fillets and coat evenly with the mixture. Now, coat each fillet with oil.
2. Arrange the fish fillets onto a greased cooking rack and spray with cooking spray. Place the drip pan in the bottom of the Instant Vortex Air Fryer Oven cooking chamber. Select "Air Fry" and then adjust the temperature to 400°F. Set the timer for 14 minutes and press "Start."

3. When the display shows "Add Food" insert the cooking rack in the center position. When the display shows "Turn Food" turn the fillets.
4. When cooking time is complete, remove the rack from the Vortex Oven. Serve hot.

Nutrition:
- Calories: 32
- Carbohydrates: 6.7 g.
- Fat: 20.3 g. Protein: 27.3 g.

98. Tuna Burgers

Preparation Time: 5 minutes
Cooking Time: 6 minutes
Servings: 4
Ingredients:
- 7 oz. canned tuna
- 1 large egg
- ¼ cup breadcrumbs
- 1 tbsp. mustard
- ¼ tsp. garlic powder
- ¼ tsp. onion powder
- ¼ tsp. cayenne pepper
- Salt and ground black pepper, as required

Directions:
1. 1 In a mixing bowl, combine all ingredients and stir until well blended. Form the ingredients into four equal-sized patties.
2. 2 Place the patties on a prepared baking sheet. Place the drip pan in the cooking chamber of the Instant Vortex Air Fryer Oven. Select "Air Fry" and set the temperature to 400°F. Set the timer for 6 minutes and hit the "Start" button.
3. 3 Place the frying rack in the center position when the display says "Add Food."
4. 4 Turn the burgers when the display says "Turn Food."
5. 5 Remove the tray from the Vortex Oven after the cooking time is over. Serve immediately.

Nutrition:
- Calories: 151
- Carbohydrates: 6.3 g.
- Fat: 6.4 g. Protein: 16.4 g.

99. Mushroom Pita Pizzas

Preparation Time: 10 minutes
Cooking Time: 5 minutes
Servings: 1
Ingredients:
- (3-inch) pitas
- 1 tablespoon olive oil
- ¾ cup pizza sauce
- 1 (4-ounce) jar sliced mushrooms, drained
- ½ teaspoon dried basil
- 2 green onions, minced
- 1 cup grated mozzarella or provolone cheese
- 1 cup sliced grape tomatoes

Directions:
1. Put each piece of pita with oil and top with the pizza sauce.
2. Put the mushrooms and sprinkle with basil and green onions. Put with the grated cheese.
3. Air fry for 5 to 10 minutes or until the cheese is melted and starts to brown. Put with the grape tomatoes.

Nutrition:
- Calories: 231 Total Fat: 9g
- Saturated Fat: 4g Cholesterol: 15mg
- Sodium: 500mg
- Carbohydrates: 25g Fiber: 2g Protein: 13g

100. Turkey Meatballs

Preparation Time: 10 minutes
Cooking Time: 20 minutes
Servings: 1
Ingredients:
- 1 lb. turkey mince
- 1 red bell pepper, deseeded and chopped
- 1 large egg, beaten
- 4 tablespoons parsley, minced
- 1 tablespoon cilantro, minced
- Salt, to taste
- Black pepper, to taste

Directions:
1. Toss all the meatball ingredients in a bowl and mix well. Make small meatballs out of this mixture and place them in the Air Fryer basket.
2. Press "Power Button" of Air Fry Oven and turn the dial to select the "Air Fry" mode. Press the Time button and again turn the dial to set the cooking time to 20 minutes
3. Now push the Temp button and rotate the dial to set the temperature at 375 degrees F. Once preheated, place the Air Fryer basket inside and close its lid. Serve warm.

Nutrition:
- Calories: 338 Fat: 9.7 g
- Carbohydrates: 32.5 g
- Protein: 10.3 g

101. English Muffin Tuna Sandwiches

Preparation Time: 8 minutes
Cooking Time: 5 minutes
Servings: 1
Ingredients:

- 1 (6-ounce) can chunk light tuna, drained
- ¼ cup mayonnaise
- Tablespoons mustard
- 1 tablespoon lemon juice
- 2 Green onions, minced
- 2 English muffins split with a fork
- 3 Tablespoons softened butter
- 2 Thin slices provolone or muenster cheese

Directions:

1. Mix the tuna, mayonnaise, mustard, lemon juice, and green onions in a small bowl.
2. Grease the cut side of the English muffins.
3. Cook butter-side up in the Air Fryer for 2 to 4 minutes or until light golden brown.
4. Take out the muffins from the Air Fryer basket.
5. Place each muffin with one slice of cheese and go back to the Air Fryer.
6. Cook for 3 to 6 minutes
7. Take out the muffins from the Air Fryer, top with the tuna mixture, and serve.

Nutrition:

- Calories: 389
- Total Fat: 23g
- Saturated Fat: 10g
- Cholesterol: 50mg
- Sodium: 495mg
- Carbohydrates: 25g
- Fiber: 3g Protein: 21g

102. Pesto Gnocchi

Preparation Time: 5 minutes
Cooking Time: 20 minutes
Servings: 1
Ingredients:

- 1 tablespoon olive oil
- 1 onion, finely chopped
- cloves garlic, sliced
- 1 (16-ounce) package shelf-stable gnocchi
- 1 (8-ounce) jar pesto
- 1 cup grated Parmesan cheese

Directions:

1. Mix the oil, onion, garlic, and gnocchi in a 6-by-6-by-2-inch pan and put it into the Air Fryer.
2. Cook for 15 minutes, then take out the pan and mix.
3. Put back the pan to the Air Fryer and cook for 13 minutes
4. Take out the pan from the Air Fryer. Place in the pesto and Parmesan cheese, and serve immediately.

Nutrition:

- Calories: 646 Total Fat: 32g
- Saturated Fat: 7g Cholesterol: 103mg
- Sodium: 461mg
- Carbohydrates: 69g Fiber: 2g
- Protein: 22g

103. Crispy Prawns

Preparation Time: 5 minutes
Cooking Time: 10 minutes
Servings: 1
Ingredients:

- 1 egg
- ½ lb. crushed nacho chips
- 12 prawns, peeled and deveined

Directions:

1. In a shallow dish, beat the egg. In another shallow dish, place the crushed nacho chips. Coat the prawn into the egg and then roll into nacho chips.
2. Arrange the coated prawns onto 2 cooking trays in a single layer. Arrange the drip pan in the bottom of the Air Fryer Oven cooking chamber. Select "Air Fry" and then adjust the temperature to 355°F. Set the time for 8 minutes and press "Start".
3. When the display shows "Add Food" insert 1 tray in the top position and another in the bottom position. When the display shows "Turn Food" do not turn the food but switch the position of cooking trays. When cooking time is complete, remove the trays from the Air Fryer oven. Serve hot.

Nutrition:

- Calories: 386 Carbohydrates: 36.1g
- Fat: 17g Protein: 21g

104. Sweet & Spicy Meatballs

Preparation Time: 20 minutes
Cooking Time: 30 minutes
Servings: 1
Ingredients:
For the meatballs:

- 2 pounds lean ground beef
- 2/3 cup quick-cooking oats

- ½ cup Ritz crackers, crushed
- 1 (5-ounce) can evaporated milk
- 2 large eggs, beaten lightly
- 1 teaspoon honey
- 1 tablespoon dried onion, minced
- 1 teaspoon garlic powder
- 1 teaspoon ground cumin
- Salt and ground black pepper, as required

For the sauce:
- 1/3 cup orange marmalade
- 1/3 cup honey
- 1/3 cup brown sugar
- 2 tablespoons cornstarch
- 2 tablespoons soy sauce
- 1-2 tablespoons hot sauce
- 1 tablespoon Worcestershire sauce

Directions:
1. For meatballs: in a large bowl, add all the ingredients and mix until well combined.
2. Make 1½-inch balls from the mixture.
3. Arrange half of the meatballs onto a cooking tray in a single layer.
4. Arrange the drip pan in the bottom of Air Fryer Oven cooking chamber.
5. Select "Air Fry" and then adjust the temperature to 380 degrees F.
6. Set the timer for 15 minutes and press the "Start".
7. When the display shows "Add Food" insert the cooking tray in the center position.
8. When the display shows "Turn Food" turn the meatballs.
9. When cooking time is complete, remove the tray from Air Fryer oven.
10. Repeat with the remaining meatballs.
11. Meanwhile, for the sauce: In a small pan, add all the ingredients over medium heat and cook until thickened, stirring continuously.
12. Serve the meatballs with the topping of sauce.

Nutrition:
- Calories: 411 Fat: 11.1 g
- Carbohydrates: 38.8 g
- Protein: 38.9 g

105. Vegetable Egg Rolls

Preparation Time: 15 minutes
Cooking Time: 10 minutes
Servings: 1
Ingredients:
- ½ Cup chopped mushrooms
- ½ cup grated carrots
- ½ cup chopped zucchini
- 2 Green onions, chopped
- 2 Tablespoons low-sodium soy sauce
- 2 Egg roll wrappers
- 1 tablespoon cornstarch
- 1 egg, beaten

Directions:
1. Mix the mushrooms, carrots, zucchini, green onions, and soy sauce, and stir together in a medium bowl.
2. Put the egg roll wrappers on a surface. Place each with about 3 tablespoons of the vegetable mixture.
3. Combine the cornstarch and egg in a small bowl.
4. Roll up the wrappers.
5. Put some of the egg mixtures on the outside of the egg rolls to seal.
6. Air fry for 8 to 10 minutes or until the egg rolls are brown and crunchy.

Nutrition:
- Calories: 112 Total Fat: 1g
- Saturated Fat: 0g Cholesterol: 23mg
- Sodium: 417mg Carbohydrates: 21g
- Fiber: 1g Protein: 4g

106. Steak With Cheese Butter

Preparation Time: 10 minutes
Cooking Time: 8 minutes
Servings: 1
Ingredients:
- 2 rib-eye steaks
- 2 teaspoon garlic powder
- 2 1/2 tbsps. blue cheese butter
- 1 teaspoon pepper
- 2 teaspoon kosher salt

Directions:
1. Preheat the Air Fryer to 400°F.
2. Mix together garlic powder, pepper, and salt and rub over the steaks.
3. Spray Air Fryer basket with cooking spray.
4. Place steak in the Air Fryer basket and cook for 4-5 minutes on each side.
5. Top with blue butter cheese.
6. Serve and enjoy.

Nutrition:
- Calories: 830 Fat: 60 g
- Carbohydrates: 3 g Sugar: 0 g
- Protein: 70g
- Cholesterol: 123 mg

107. Potatoes with Black Beans

Preparation Time: 6 minutes
Cooking Time: 18 minutes
Servings: 3
Ingredients:
- 1 potato, mashed
- 1 can black beans
- 1 tbsp. lime juice
- 2 garlic cloves, minced
- 1/3 cup cheddar cheese, shredded
- Salt to taste

Directions:
1. Make a layer of mashed potato in the round baking dish.
2. Add black beans, lime juice, garlic, and salt.
3. Sprinkle cheese to cover the mixture.
4. Place the tray in the Air Fryer to cook for 18 minutes at 300°F.
5. When done, serve!

Nutrition:
- Calories: 75
- Sodium: 767mg
- Protein: 100g
- Carbohydrates: 20g
- Fat: 9g
- Potassium: 968mg

108. Lentils with Mushrooms

Preparation Time: 6 minutes
Cooking Time: 20 minutes
Servings: 3
Ingredients:
- 1 tbsp. oil
- 2 white onions, sliced
- 3 garlic cloves, minced
- ½ cup lentils
- 2 cups water
- 3 cups mushrooms
- Salt to taste
- 1 tsp. cumin powder
- Black pepper to taste

Directions:
1. Grease oil in the baking tray.
2. Add onion, garlic, and then the lentils.
3. Add water and let it cook for 10 minutes in the Air Fryer at 300°F.
4. Add mushrooms with cumin powder, black pepper, and salt according to your taste.
5. Cook for another 10 minutes.
6. When ready, serve immediately and enjoy!

Nutrition:
- Calories: 75 Sodium: 106.7mg
- Protein: 100g Carbohydrates: 20g
- Fat: 9g Potassium: 637.4mg

109. Quick Eggplant Air Fryer Recipe

Preparation Time: 4 minutes
Cooking Time: 16 minutes
Servings: 2
Ingredients:
- 2 large eggplants
- Salt to taste
- 1/3 cup oil
- 1 tbsp. honey–
- 1 tsp. paprika
- ½ tsp. cumin powder
- 4 garlic cloves, chopped
- 1 lemon juice
- 1 tbsp. soy sauce
- 1 bunch parsley
- 2 oz cheese

Directions:
1. Grease oil in the baking tray.
2. Mix salt, honey, paprika, cumin powder, garlic cloves, lemon juice, soy sauce and parsley in a bowl.
3. Place the eggplants in the baking tray and pour the mixture as well.
4. Spread cheese on the entire mixture.
5. Place the tray in the Air Fryer for 16 minutes on 300°F.
6. When ready, serve and enjoy!

Nutrition:
- Calories: 90
- Sodium: 960mg
- Protein: 270g
- Carbohydrates: 10g
- Fat: 4g
- Potassium: 417mg

110. Chicken and Avocado Recipes

Preparation Time: 6 minutes
Cooking Time: 15 minutes
Servings: 3
Ingredients:
- ½ cup red onion, chopped
- 1 bunch cilantro, chopped
- 1 jalapeno, minced
- 1 tbsp. lime juice
- 2 garlic cloves, minced

- 4 tomatoes, diced
- 4 avocados, cubed
- 1 lb. boneless chicken, cubes

Directions:
1. Add chicken to the round baking tray along with lime juice.
2. Let it cook in the Air Fryer for 10 minutes at 300°F.
3. Add red onion, cilantro, jalapeno, garlic, tomatoes, and avocados on top of the chicken.
4. Cook for another 15 minutes.
5. When ready, serve!

Nutrition:
- Calories: 92
- Sodium: 109.4 mg
- Protein: 108g
- Carbohydrates: 45g
- Fat: 11g Potassium: 911mg

111. Grounded Chicken with Mushrooms

Preparation Time: 5 minutes
Cooking Time: 10 minutes
Servings: 3
Ingredients:
- 1 lb. grounded Chicken
- 4 oz Mushrooms, chopped
- ½ onion, diced
- 3 garlic cloves, minced
- 2 green onions, chopped
- 1 bunch cilantro, chopped
- 1 Lemon, juice
- 1 tsp. garlic sauce
- 1 tbsp. olive oil
- 1 bunch lettuce
- 1 avocado, sliced

Directions:
1. Grease the round baking tray with oil.
2. Add the minced garlic along with the chicken. Stir it well, so the chicken cooks and gets soft to eat.
3. Add lemon juice and stir it well.
4. Add soy sauce, chili sauce, cilantro, and green onions.
5. Mix it well and let it cook in the Air Fryer at 300°F for 10 minutes.
6. When cooked, pour it into a bowl and dress it with onions and lettuce on the top with avocado slices.
7. Chop the mushrooms and sprinkle them as a last layer. Enjoy eating when ready!

Nutrition:
- Calories: 92 Sodium: 606mg
- Protein: 108g
- Carbohydrates: 45g
- Fat: 11g Potassium: 829mg

112. Chicken with Avocado Mix

Preparation Time: 6 minutes
Cooking Time: 14 minutes
Servings: 2
Ingredients:
- 2 cups chicken
- ½ avocado, sliced
- Salt and pepper to taste
- 2 radish, sliced
- Parsley, chopped, for dressing

Directions:
1. Cut the chicken into slices and add it to the bowl.
2. Slice the radish and cut the avocado by placing it on top of the chicken. When done, dress it with parsley and mix.
3. Add it to the round baking tray and place it in the Air Fryer.
4. Let it cook for 14 minutes at 300°F.
5. When ready, add salt and pepper at the end to enjoy the salad.

Nutrition:
- Calories: 90 Sodium: 235mg
- Protein: 110g
- Carbohydrates: 45g Fat: 16g
- Potassium: 677mg

113. Eggs with Vegs

Preparation Time: 4 minutes
Cooking Time: 6 minutes
Servings: 2
Ingredients:
- 2 eggs, boiled
- ½ onion, chopped
- 6 celery, cut
- 2 cups dill pickles, diced
- 1 cup Mayo
- 1 tsp. yellow mustard
- 1 cup cheese, shredded
- Salt and pepper to taste

Directions:
1. Chop the boiled eggs and add them to a bowl.

2. Now add onions, celery, dill pickles, yellow mustard, and mayo. Mix it well together.
3. Pour the mixture into the round baking tray and cover it with shredded cheese.
4. Place it in the Air Fryer for 6 minutes at 300°F.
5. Add salt and pepper as desired. When ready, eat and enjoy!

Nutrition:
- Calories: 75
- Sodium: 510mg
- Protein: 100g
- Carbohydrates: 20g
- Fat: 9g
- Potassium: 322mg

114. Chicken with Lettuce

Preparation Time: 5 minutes
Cooking Time: 15 minutes
Servings: 3
Ingredients:
- 12 oz chicken breast, sliced
- 3 garlic cloves, chopped
- 1 cup avocado, chopped
- 1 red onion, diced
- 6 cups lettuce, chopped
- 2 tbsp. olive oil
- 2 tbsp. balsamic vinegar
- Pepper to taste

Directions:
1. Add chicken to the round baking tray with garlic. Place it in the Air Fryer for 15 minutes at 300°F.
2. When ready, cut the chicken into slices.
3. Add the chicken along with the avocado, red onion, lettuce, olive oil, balsamic vinegar, and pepper in a bowl.
4. Mix it well and gently.
5. When ready, enjoy it with your friends and family.

Nutrition:
- Calories: 92 Sodium: 437mg
- Protein: 108G Carbohydrates: 45g
- Fat: 11g
- Potassium: 734mg

115. Bacon with Vegetables

Preparation Time: 6 minutes
Cooking Time: 15 minutes
Servings: 3
Ingredients:
- 5 bacon slices
- 1 ½ tsp. oil–
- 1 lime, juice
- 1/3 cup soy sauce
- 2 garlic cloves, minced
- 2 tsp. red pepper flakes
- 1 cup carrots, grated
- ¼ cup peanuts, chopped
- ½ cup cilantro, chopped

Directions:
1. Grease oil in the round baking tray.
2. Add lime juice, soy sauce, garlic, red pepper flakes, carrots and peanuts.
3. Place the bacon slices over it.
4. Cook in the Air Fryer for 15 minutes at 300°F.
5. When done, garnish with parsley and enjoy!

Nutrition:
- Calories: 90
- Sodium: 284mg
- Protein: 257g
- Carbohydrates: 10g
- Fat: 4g
- Potassium: 69.7mg

116. Avocado with Eggs

Preparation Time: 6 minutes
Cooking Time: 10 minutes
Servings: 2
Ingredients:
- 1 avocado, chopped
- 2 eggs boiled, chopped
- 1 tomato, chopped
- 1 tbsp. lemon juice
- Salt and pepper to taste
- Parsley to garnish

Directions:
1. Get the round baking tray and place the chopped boiled eggs as a layer.
2. Add avocado, boiled eggs, tomato, and lemon juice.
3. Mix it well and add salt and pepper as desired. Cook in the Air Fryer for 10 minutes at 300°F.
4. When ready, garnish it with chopped parsley.
5. Serve and enjoy the dish!

Nutrition:
- Calories: 90 Sodium: 360mg
- Protein: 110g Carbohydrates: 45g
- Fat: 16g Potassium: 627mg

117. Beef Steak Air Fryer

Preparation Time: 4 minutes
Cooking Time: 18 minutes
Servings: 3
Ingredients:
- 1/4 cup balsamic Vinegar
- 1/2 cup Soy sauce
- 2 tsp. Worcestershire sauce
- 1/2 tsp. onion powder
- 1/2 tsp. smoke flavor liquid
- 2 garlic cloves, chopped
- 1/2 tbsp. honey
- 1 tbsp. olive oil
- Salt and pepper to taste
- 2 pinches Cayenne pepper
- 3 Beef Steak

Directions:
1. Grease oil in the baking tray.
2. Mix Worcestershire sauce, salt and pepper, honey, cayenne pepper, garlic, soy sauce, olive oil, onion powder, and liquid smoke flavor by adding vinegar at the end. Stir well.
3. Now cover the beef with the sauce in the tray.
4. Place it in the Air Fryer for 18 minutes.
5. Let it cook at 350°F.
6. When ready, serve!

Nutrition:
- Calories: 75
- Sodium: 4043mg
- Protein: 100g
- Carbohydrates: 20g
- Fat: 9g
- Potassium: 660.8mg

118. Chicken Breast Air Fryer

Preparation Time: 6 minutes
Cooking Time: 15 minutes
Servings: 2
Ingredients:
- 2 tbsp. olive oil
- 2 tbsp. onion, chopped
- 2 garlic cloves, chopped
- 1/2 tsp. thyme, dried
- Salt and pepper to taste
- 1/3 tsp. hot pepper sauce
- 3 pieces chicken breast
- 1 bunch parsley
- 1 tsp. rosemary, dried
- 1 tsp. sage, powder
- 1/3 tsp. Marjoram, dried

Directions:
1. Grease oil in the baking tray.
2. Mix sage, thyme, salt and pepper, marjoram, rosemary, sage, onion, and hot pepper sauce together. Stir well.
3. Now cover the chicken in the sauce and place the tray in the Air Fryer.
4. Let it cook for 15 minutes at 300°F.
5. When done, serve and enjoy the meal.

Nutrition:
- Calories: 29
- Sodium: 515mg
- Protein: 140g
- Carbohydrates: 45g
- Fat: 36g
- Potassium: 967mg

119. Delicious Chicken

Preparation Time: 6 minutes
Cooking Time: 10 minutes
Servings: 3
Ingredients:
- 1 lb. boneless chicken
- 1 lettuce, chopped
- 1 tomato, chopped
- ½ cup Cheese, low-fat
- 3 bacon slices
- 2 eggs, boiled
- Ranch dressing (optional)
- Pepper to taste
- A bunch parsley, chopped

Directions:
1. Add chicken to the round baking tray.
2. Add lettuce, tomato, cheese, eggs, pepper, and parsley. Mix well.
3. Now cut the bacon slices into pieces and spread them over the mixture.
4. Place the tray in the Air Fryer for 10 minutes on 300°F.
5. When ready, enjoy!

Nutrition:
- Calories: 90
- Sodium: 1045mg
- Protein: 257g
- Carbohydrates: 10g
- Fat: 4g
- Potassium: 438mg

120. Simple Asparagus Treat

Preparation Time: 6 minutes
Cooking Time: 16 minutes
Servings: 2
Ingredients:

- 2 lbs. asparagus
- 1 tbsp. butter
- 1 onion, chopped
- 6 cups chicken broth
- 2 tbsp. sour cream, low-fat
- Salt and pepper to taste

Directions:

1. Butter the round baking tray.
2. Add onion, chicken broth, sour cream and salt, and pepper with asparagus.
3. Place the tray in the Air Fryer.
4. Let it cook for 16 minutes at 300°F.
5. When ready, serve and enjoy!

Nutrition:

- Calories: 75
- Sodium: 3.6mg
- Protein: 100g
- Carbohydrates: 20g
- Fat: 9g
- Potassium: 270.3mg

121. Eggs with Carrots and Peas

Preparation Time: 5 minutes
Cooking Time: 20 minutes
Servings: 2
Ingredients:

- 2 cups peas
- 1/2 cup olive oil
- 2 Onions, sliced
- 2 carrots, chopped
- 2 Garlic cloves, minced
- 1 cauliflower
- 2 tbsp. soy sauce
- 2 Eggs

Directions:

1. Whisk the eggs into a bowl and keep them aside.
2. Grease oil in the round baking tray.
3. Add the peas, carrots, onions, and cauliflower to the tray.
4. Mix minced garlic cloves with soy sauce.
5. Pour the egg and place the tray in the Air Fryer.
6. Let it cook for 20 minutes at 300°F.
7. When ready, serve and enjoy the meal!

Nutrition:

- Calories: 90
- Sodium: 156mg
- Protein: 110g
- Carbohydrates: 45g
- Fat: 16g
- Potassium: 189mg

CHAPTER 10:

Vegetarian Recipes

122. Delicious Air Fryer Cauliflower

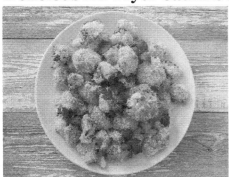

Preparation Time: 5 minutes
Cooking Time: 10 minutes
Servings: 6
Ingredients:

- 1/2 tsp fresh lemon juice
- 3 cups cauliflower
- Salt and pepper to taste (very little)
- 1 tbsp fresh parsley, chopped
- ¾ tsp dried oregano
- 1 1/2 tsp olive oil
- 1 tbsp pine nuts (unsalted)

Directions:

1. Place the cauliflower in a container and sprinkle it with olive oil. Add oregano, salt, and pepper.
2. Place in the fryer at 375°F and fry for 10 minutes.
3. Drop into a serving dish and include pine nuts, fresh parsley, and lemon juice.

Nutrition:

- Calories: 104
- Fat: 7 g
- Carbohydrates: 9 g
- Protein: 44 g

123. Spinach Quiche

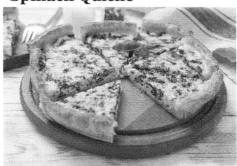

Preparation Time: 10 minutes
Cooking Time: 18/22 minutes
Servings: 3
Ingredients:

- 3 eggs
- 1 cup frozen chopped spinach, thawed and drained
- 1/3 cup heavy cream
- 2 tablespoons honey mustard
- 1/2 cup grated Swiss or Havarti cheese
- 1/2 teaspoon dried thyme
- Pinch salt (very little)
- Freshly ground black pepper, to taste (very little)
- Nonstick baking spray with flour

Directions:

1. In a medium bowl, beat the eggs until blended. Add the spinach, cream, honey mustard, cheese, thyme, salt and pepper and mix evenly.
2. Spray a fryer basket or fryer-friendly pan with nonstick spray. Pour the egg mixture inside.
3. Cook for 18-22 minutes in the Air Fryer at 380°F or until the egg mixture is puffed, lightly golden and set.
4. Let cool for 5 minutes, then cut into wedges to serve.

Nutrition:

- Calories: 203 Total Fat: 15 g
- Carbohydrates: 6 g
- Protein: 71 g

124. Yellow Squash Fritters

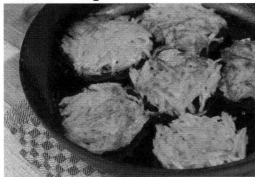

Preparation Time: 15 minutes
Cooking Time: 7/9 minutes
Servings: 4
Ingredients:

- 1 (3-ounce) package cream cheese, softened
- 1 egg, beaten
- 1/2 teaspoon dried oregano
- Pinch salt (very little)
- Freshly ground black pepper, to taste (very little)
- 1 medium yellow summer squash, grated
- 1/3 cup grated carrot
- 2/3 cup bread crumbs
- 2 tablespoons olive oil

Directions:

1. In a medium bowl, combine and mix well the cream cheese with the egg, oregano, salt, and pepper. Add the pumpkin and the carrot and mix well. Add the breadcrumbs and mix well.
2. Form about 2 tablespoons of this mixture into a patty about 1/2 inch thick. Repeat with the remaining mixture. Brush pancakes with olive oil.
3. Air-fry until crisp and golden at 380°F, about 7 to 9 minutes.

Nutrition:

- Calories: 134
- Total Fat: 17 g
- Carbohydrates: 16 g
- Protein: 56 g

125. Eggplant Parmigiana

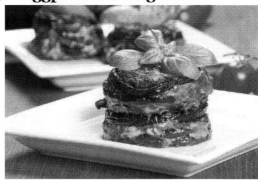

Preparation Time: 15 minutes
Cooking Time: 20 minutes
Servings: 4
Ingredients:

- 1 medium eggplant (about 1-pound), sliced into 1/2-inch-thick rounds
- 2 tablespoons tamari or shoyu
- 3 tablespoons non-dairy milk, plain and unsweetened
- 1 cup chickpea flour
- 1 tablespoon dried basil
- 1 tablespoon dried oregano
- 2 teaspoons garlic granules
- 2 teaspoons onion granules
- 1/2 teaspoon sea salt
- 1/2 teaspoon freshly ground black pepper
- Cooking oil spray (sunflower or safflower)
- Vegan marinara sauce, to taste (your choice)
- Shredded cheese, to taste (preferably mozzarella)

Directions:

1. Place the eggplant slices in a large bowl, and pour the tamari and milk over the top. Turn the pieces over to coat them as evenly as possible with the liquids. Set aside.
2. In a medium bowl, combine the flour, basil, oregano, garlic, onion, salt, and pepper and stir well. Set aside.
3. Spray the Air Fryer basket with oil and set it aside.
4. Stir the eggplant slices again and transfer them to a plate (stacking is fine). Do not discard the liquid in the bowl.
5. Bread the eggplant by tossing an eggplant round in the flour mixture. Then, dip in the liquid again. Double up on the coating by placing the eggplant again in the flour mixture, making sure that all sides are nicely breaded. Place in the Air Fryer basket.

6. Repeat with enough eggplant rounds to make a (mostly) single layer in the Air Fryer basket. (You'll need to cook it in batches so that you don't have too much overlap and it cooks perfectly.)
7. Spray the tops of the eggplant with enough oil so that you no longer see dry patches in the coating. Fry for 8 minutes at 385°F. Remove the Air Fryer basket and spray the tops again. Turn each piece over, again taking care not to overlap the rounds too much. Spray the tops with oil, again making sure that no dry patches remain. Fry for another 8 minutes, or until nicely browned and crisp. Repeat until all eggplant is crisp and golden brown. Finally, place half of the eggplant in a 6-inch round baking dish, 2 inches deep, and cover with the marinara sauce and a sprinkling of vegan cheese. Fry for 3 minutes, or until the sauce is hot and the cheese is melted (be careful not to overcook, or the edges of the eggplant will burn). Serve immediately, plain or over pasta.

Nutrition:
- Calories: 217 Total fat: 9 g
- Carbohydrates: 38 g Protein: 69 g

126. Air Fryer Brussels Sprouts

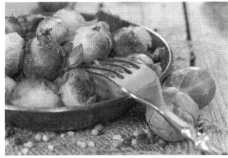

Preparation Time: 10 minutes
Cooking Time: 8/12 minutes
Servings: 2
Ingredients:
- 1 cup brussels sprouts
- 1/4 cup balsamic vinegar
- 3 tbsp. extra-virgin olive oil
- Kosher salt to taste (very little)
- Freshly ground black pepper to taste (very little)

Directions:
1. Remove hard ends of Brussels sprouts and discard damaged outer leaves. Rinse under cold water and pat dry. If your sprouts are large, cut them in half. Add and season with oil, salt and pepper.
2. Arrange the Brussels sprouts in a single layer in the Air Fryer and work in batches if they don't all fit. Bake for 8-12 minutes at 190°C and shake the pan halfway through to brown them evenly. They're ready when they're lightly browned and crispy at the edges.
3. Serve the sprouts warm, optionally with a balsamic reduction and parmesan cheese.

Nutrition:
- Calories: 164
- Protein: 69.58 g
- Fat: 15.97 g
- Carbohydrates: 16.97 g

127. Endives with Bacon Mix

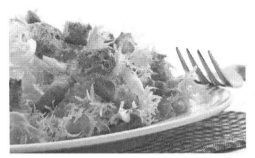

Preparation Time: 15 minutes
Cooking Time: 10 minutes
Servings: 1
Ingredients:
- 4 endives, trimmed and halved
- Salt and black pepper to taste (very little)
- 1 tbsp. olive oil
- 2 tbsp. bacon, cooked and crumbled
- 1/2 tsp. nutmeg, ground

Directions:
1. Place the endives in your Air Fryer's basket, then add the salt and pepper to taste as well as oil and nutmeg ensure to toss gently.
2. Cook at a temperature of 360°F for 10 minutes.
3. Cut the endives into different plates, then sprinkle the bacon as toppings, and serve.

Nutrition:
- Calories: 151
- Fat: 6
- Carbohydrates: 14
- Protein: 66

128. Creamy Potatoes

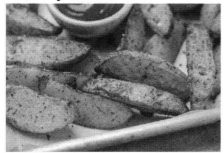

Preparation Time: 10 minutes
Cooking Time: 20 minutes
Servings: 1
Ingredients:

- ¾ pound potatoes, peeled and cubed
- 1 tablespoon olive oil
- Salt and black pepper, to taste (very little)
- 1/2 cup Greek yogurt

Directions:

1. Place potatoes in a bowl, pour water to cover, and leave aside for 10 minutes.
2. Drain, pat dry, and then transfer to another bowl.
3. Add salt, pepper, and half of the oil to the potatoes and mix.
4. Put potatoes in the Air Fryer basket and cook at 360ºF for 20 minutes.
5. In a bowl, mix yogurt with salt, pepper, and the rest of the oil and whisk.
6. Divide potatoes onto plates, drizzle with yogurt dressing, mix, and serve.

Nutrition:

- Calories: 170
- Fat: 3 g
- Carbohydrates: 20 g
- Protein: 75 g

129. Creamy Cabbage

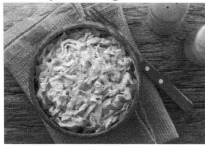

Preparation Time: 10 minutes
Cooking Time: 20 minutes
Servings: 1
Ingredients:

- 1/2 green cabbage head, chopped
- 1/2 yellow onion, chopped
- Salt and black pepper, to taste (very little)
- 1/2 cup whipped cream
- 1 tablespoon cornstarch

Directions:

1. Put cabbage and onion in the Air Fryer.
2. In a bowl, mix cornstarch with cream, salt, and pepper. Stir and pour over cabbage.
3. Mix well and then bake at 400ºF for 20 minutes.
4. Serve.

Nutrition:

- Calories: 208
- Fat: 10 g
- Carbohydrates: 16 g
- Protein: 55 g

130. Asparagus & Parmesan

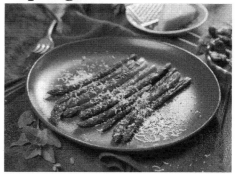

Preparation Time: 10 minutes
Cooking Time: 6 minutes
Servings: 1
Ingredients:

- 1 teaspoon sesame oil
- 11 oz asparagus
- 1 teaspoon chicken stock
- 1/2 teaspoon ground white pepper
- 3 oz Parmesan

Directions:

1. Wash the asparagus and chop it roughly.
2. Sprinkle the chopped asparagus with the chicken stock and ground white pepper.
3. Then sprinkle the asparagus with the sesame oil and shake them.
4. Place the asparagus in the Air Fryer basket.
5. Cook them for 4 minutes at 400ºF.
6. Meanwhile, shred Parmesan cheese.
7. When the time is over shaking the asparagus gently and sprinkle with the shredded cheese.
8. Cook the asparagus for 2 minutes more at 400ºF.

9. After this, transfer the cooked asparagus to the serving plates.

Nutrition:
- Calories: 139
- Fat: 11.6 g
- Carbohydrates: 7.9 g
- Protein: 57.2 g

131. Walnut & Cheese Filled Mushrooms

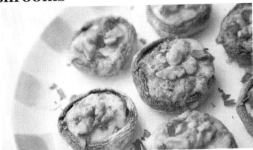

Preparation Time: 5 minutes
Cooking Time: 10 minutes
Servings: 1
Ingredients:
- 4 large Portobello mushroom caps
- 1/3 cup walnuts, minced
- 1 tbsp canola oil
- 1/2 cup mozzarella cheese, shredded
- 1 tbsp fresh parsley, chopped
- Cooking Spray

Directions:
1. Preheat the Air Fryer to 350°F. Grease the Air Fryer basket with cooking spray.
2. Rub the mushrooms with canola oil and fill them with mozzarella cheese. Top with minced walnuts and arrange on the bottom of the greased Air Fryer basket.
3. Bake for 10 minutes to 350°F or until golden on top. Remove, let cool for a few minutes and sprinkle with freshly chopped parsley to serve.

Nutrition:
- Calories: 110
- Carbohydrates: 6 g
- Fat: 5 g
- Protein: 78 g

132. Chard with Cheddar

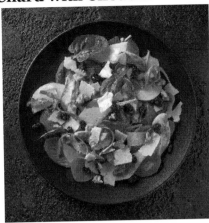

Preparation Time: 10 minutes
Cooking Time: 11 minutes
Servings: 1
Ingredients:
- 3 oz Cheddar cheese, grated
- 10 oz Swiss chard
- 3 tablespoons cream
- 1 tablespoon sesame oil
- Salt and pepper to taste (very little)

Directions:
1. Wash Swiss chard carefully and chop it roughly.
2. Sprinkle the chopped chard with salt and ground pepper.
3. Stir it carefully.
4. Sprinkle Swiss chard with the sesame oil and stir it carefully with the help of 2 spatulas.
5. Preheat the Air Fryer to 260°F.
6. Put chopped Swiss chard in the Air Fryer basket and cook for 6 minutes.
7. Shake it after 3 minutes of cooking.
8. Then pour the cream into the Air Fryer basket and mix it up.
9. Cook for 3 minutes more.
10. Then increase the temperature to 400°F.
11. Sprinkle with the grated cheese and bake for another 2 minutes.
12. After this, transfer the meal to the serving plates. Enjoy!

Nutrition:
- Calories: 172
- Fat: 22.3 g
- Carbohydrates: 6.7 g
- Protein: 63.3 g

133. Herbed Tomatoes

Preparation Time: 10 minutes
Cooking Time: 15 minutes
Servings: 1
Ingredients:

- 2 big tomatoes, halved and insides scooped out
- Salt and black pepper, to taste (very little)
- 1/2 tablespoon olive oil
- 1 garlic clove, minced
- 1/4 teaspoon thyme, chopped

Directions:

1. In the Air Fryer, mix tomatoes with thyme, garlic, oil, salt, and pepper.
2. Mix and cook at 390°F for 15 minutes.
3. Serve.

Nutrition:

- Calories: 112 Fat: 1 g
- Carbohydrates: 4 g Protein: 34 g

134. Spiced Almonds

Preparation Time: 5 minutes
Cooking Time: 12 minutes
Servings: 1
Ingredients:

- 1/2 tsp ground cinnamon
- 1 cup almonds
- 1 egg white
- Sea salt to taste (very little)
- Cooking Spray

Directions:

1. Preheat the Air Fryer to 310°F.
2. Grease the Air Fryer basket with cooking spray.
3. Take a bowl and split the egg whites of the eggs, being careful of the egg skin chips and removing them if necessary.
4. In another bowl, whisk the egg white with cinnamon and the almonds and mix well to flavor the almonds with the egg white and spices.
5. Spread the almonds on the bottom of the frying basket and Air-fry for 12 minutes to 310°F, shaking once or twice. Remove and sprinkle with sea salt to serve.

Nutrition:

- Calories: 90
- Carbohydrates: 3 g
- Fat: 2 g
- Protein: 45 g

135. Leeks

Preparation Time: 10 minutes
Cooking Time: 7 minutes
Servings: 1
Ingredients:

- 2 leeks, washed, ends cut, and halved
- Salt and black pepper, to taste (very little)
- 1/2 tablespoon butter, melted
- 1/2 tablespoon lemon juice

Directions:

1. Season leeks with melted butter and season with salt and pepper.
2. Lay it inside the Air Fryer and cook at 350°F for 7 minutes.
3. Arrange on a platter.
4. Drizzle with lemon juice and serve.

Nutrition:

- Calories: 100 Fat: 4 g
- Carbohydrates: 6 g
- Protein: 32 g

136. Asparagus

Preparation Time: 5 minutes
Cooking Time: 8 minutes
Servings: 1
Ingredients:

- Nutritional yeast, to taste
- Olive oil nonstick spray
- 1 bunch of asparagus

Directions:

1. Wash asparagus and then trim off thick, woody ends.
2. Spray asparagus with olive oil spray and sprinkle with yeast.
3. Add the asparagus to the basket of the Air Fryer in a single layer. Set the temperature to 360°F and set the time to 8 minutes.
4. Remove them from the fryer and serve.

Nutrition:

- Calories: 17
- Total Fat: 8 g
- Total Carbohydrates: 2 g
- Protein: 39 g

137. Lemony Lentils with "Fried" Onions

Preparation Time: 10 minutes
Cooking Time: 30/35 minutes
Servings: 4
Ingredients:

- 1 cup red lentils

- 4 cups water
- Cooking oil spray (sunflower or safflower)
- 1 medium-size onion, peeled and cut into 1/4-inch-thick rings
- 1/2 cup kale, stems removed, thinly sliced
- 3 large garlic cloves, pressed or minced
- 2 tablespoons fresh lemon juice
- 2 teaspoons nutritional yeast
- 1/2 teaspoon sea salt
- 1 teaspoon lemon zest
- ¾ teaspoon freshly ground black pepper

Directions:
1. In a medium saucepan, place the lentils with the water on the stove and simmer uncovered until the lentils have completely dissolved, about 30 minutes. Stir every 5 minutes or so while cooking so the lentils don't stick to the bottom of the pot.
2. While the lentils are cooking spray the Air Fryer basket with oil and place the onion rings inside, separating them as much as possible spray them with the oil and sprinkle with a little salt.
3. Then fry for 5 minutes and remove the Air Fryer basket, stir and spray again with oil.
4. Fry for another 5 minutes.
5. All of the onion slices to be crisp and well browned, so if some of the pieces begin to do that, transfer them from the Air Fryer basket to a plate.
6. Remove the Air Fryer basket and spray the onions again with oil. Fry for another 5 minutes or until all the pieces are crisp and browned.
7. Add the kale to the hot lentils and stir very well to finish the lentils.
8. Stir in the garlic, Nutrition yeast, lemon juice, zest, salt, and pepper.
9. Stir very well, distribute evenly in bowls and top with the crisp onion rings.

Nutrition:
- Calories: 120
- Total fat: 1 g
- Carbohydrates: 39 g
- Protein: 85 g

138. Cauliflower Steak

Preparation Time: 12 minutes
Cooking Time: 7 minutes
Servings: 1
Ingredients:
- 1 medium head cauliflower
- 1/4 cup blue cheese crumbles
- 1/4 cup full-fat ranch dressing (not spicy)
- 1 tbsp. Salted butter melted.

Directions:
1. Remove cauliflower leaves and slice the head in 1/2-inch-thick slices.
2. In a small bowl, mix hot sauce with butter and brush the mixture over the cauliflower.
3. Place each cauliflower steak into the Air Fryer and set the temperature to 400°F. Cook for 7 minutes.
4. When cooked, edges will begin turning dark and caramelized. Sprinkle steaks with crumbled blue cheese and serve. Drizzle with ranch dressing.

Nutrition:
- Calories: 122
- Protein: 54.9 g
- Fat: 8.4 g
- Carbohydrates: 7.7 g

139. Onion Green Beans

Preparation Time: 10 minutes
Cooking Time: 12 minutes
Servings: 1
Ingredients:
- 11 oz green beans
- 1 tablespoon onion powder
- 1 tablespoon olive oil
- 1/2 teaspoon salt

Directions:
1. Wash the green beans carefully and place them in the bowl.
2. Sprinkle the green beans with onion powder, salt, and olive oil.
3. Shake the green beans carefully.
4. Preheat the Air Fryer to 400°F.
5. Put the green beans in the Air Fryer and cook for 8 minutes.
6. After this, shake the green beans and cook them for 4 minutes more at 400°F.
7. When the time is over shaking the green beans.
8. Serve the side dish and enjoy!

Nutrition:
- Calories: 175
- Fat: 7.2 g
- Carbohydrates: 13.9 g
- Protein: 63.2 g

140. Green Beans and Cherry Tomatoes

Preparation Time: 10 minutes
Cooking Time: 15 minutes
Servings: 1
Ingredients:

- 8 oz cherry tomatoes
- 8 oz green beans
- 1 tablespoon olive oil
- Salt and black pepper, to taste (very little)

Directions:

1. In a bowl, mix cherry tomatoes with green beans, olive oil, salt, and pepper. Mix.
2. Cook in the Air Fryer at 400°F for 15 minutes. Shake once.
3. Serve.

Nutrition:

- Calories: 162
- Fat: 6 g
- Carbohydrates: 8 g
- Protein: 89 g

141. Onion Soup

Preparation Time: 5 minutes
Cooking Time: 35 minutes
Servings: 1
Ingredients:

- 2 large white onions, peeled, sliced
- ½ cup cubed squash
- 1 sprig of thyme
- 1 tbsp. grapeseed oil
- 2 cups spring water

Extra:

- ½ teaspoon salt
- ¼ teaspoon cayenne pepper

Directions:

1. Take a medium pot, place it over medium heat, add oil, and when hot, add onion and cook for 10 minutes.
2. Add thyme sprig, switch heat to the low level and then cook onions for 15 to 20 minutes until soft, covering the pan with its lid.
3. Add the remaining ingredients, stir until mixed and simmer for 5 minutes.
4. Ladle soup into bowls and then serve.

Nutrition:

- Calories: 76 Carbohydrates: 13.1 g
- Protein: 2.3 g
- Fat: 2.1 g

142. Basil Parmesan Tomatoes

Preparation Time: 30 minutes
Cooking Time: 20 minutes
Servings: 1
Ingredients:

- ½ teaspoon dried oregano
- 4 roam tomatoes
- Spices: onion powder, garlic powder, sea salt, and black pepper
- ½ cup parmesan cheese, shredded
- 12 small fresh basil leaves

Directions:

1. Preheat the oven to 425°F and grease a baking sheet lightly. Mix together dried oregano, onion powder, garlic powder, sea salt, and black pepper in a small bowl.
2. Arrange the tomato slices on a baking sheet and sprinkle with the seasoning blend. Top with parmesan cheese and basil leaves and transfer to the oven. Bake for about 20 min and remove from the oven to servings.

Nutrition:

- Calories: 49
- Carbohydrates: 4.3 g
- Protein: 3.9 g
- Fat: 2.2 g

143. Beef Chop Salad

Preparation Time: 15 minutes
Cooking Time: 0 minutes
Servings: 1
Ingredients:

- 1 medium English cucumber, chopped (2 cups)
- 1 cup halved cherry tomatoes
- 1 red bell pepper, seeded and diced
- ½ red onion, diced
- ½ cup pitted kalamata olives, roughly chopped
- 1 cup crumbled feta cheese
- ½ cup balsamic dressing

Directions:

1. In a large bowl, toss the cucumber, tomatoes, bell pepper, onion, olives, and cheese with the dressing, and servings.

Ingredient tip: looking for a protein boost? Add diced chicken breast or chickpeas.

Nutrition:

- Calories: 173 Carbohydrates: 10 g
- Protein: 4 g
- Fat: 13 g

144. Roasted Veggies

Preparation Time: 5 minutes
Cooking Time: 30 minutes
Servings: 1
Ingredients:
- 1 medium bell pepper, cut into strips
- 1 small onion, halved then sliced
- 1 small zucchini, sliced into rounds
- 2 tbsps. extra-virgin olive oil
- Salt to taste - 1-pint grape tomatoes
- Freshly ground black pepper

Directions:
2. Preheat the oven to 400°F.
3. Using 1 or 2 large baking sheets, arrange the vegetables so they are lying flat, lightly touching each other.
4. Evenly pour the olive oil over the vegetables, and gently toss to coat, using either a spoon or your hands. Add salt and pepper to taste.
5. Roast for 20 to 30 min, or until soft and lightly charred, stirring halfway through, and servings.

Nutrition:
- Calories: 75 Carbohydrates: 8 g
- Protein: 0 g Fat: 5 g

145. Cabbage Salad

Preparation Time: 10 minutes
Cooking Time: 15 minutes
Servings: 1
Ingredients:
- 2 ½ cup Cabbage (shredded)
- 1 tsp. Salt
- Low-fat mayonnaise (as needed to coat)

Directions:
1. Mix all ingredients together.

Nutrition:
- Calories: 55
- Carbohydrates: 2 g
- Protein: 1 g
- Fat: 1 g

146. Potato Salad

Preparation Time: 20 minutes
Cooking Time: 1 hours
Servings: 1
Ingredients:
- 3 cups Potatoes (cubed, boiled, cold)
- 1 tsp. Onion (finely chopped)
- Salt (dash)
- Black pepper (dash)
- Pimiento (to taste, optional)
- Parsley (to taste, optional)
- ½ cup French dressing
- ¾ cup Low-fat mayonnaise

Directions:
2. Boil the eggs. Let cool. Chill.
3. Peel, cube, and boil the potatoes until soft but not falling apart. Cool.
4. Chop the onions.
5. Put the cooled potatoes and the onions together in a bowl.
6. Season with salt and pepper. Mix gently.
7. Add the French dressing. Mix gently. Chill 1-2 hours.
8. Add the mayonnaise, pimiento and parsley. Mix gently.
9. Dice and add the chilled eggs. Mix gently.
10. Add extra seasonings to taste.
11. Dish up into individual bowls. For more variety, place on individual plates surrounded with salad greens, cucumber sticks, slices of boiled eggs, and/or tomato pieces.

Nutrition:
- Calories: 74
- Carbohydrates: 2 g
- Protein: 1 g
- Fat: 1 g

147. Spaghetti Squash Chow Mein

Preparation Time: 10 minutes
Cooking Time: 55 minutes
Servings: 1
Ingredients:
- Nonstick cooking spray
- 1 small (3- to 4-pound) spaghetti squash
- ¼ cup low-sodium soy sauce
- 3 garlic cloves, minced
- 1 tablespoon oyster sauce
- 1-inch ginger root, peeled and minced
- 2 tablespoons extra-virgin olive oil
- 1 small white onion, diced
- 3 celery stalks, thinly sliced
- 2 cups shredded cabbage (or coleslaw mix)

Directions:

1. Preheat the oven to 350°F. Coat a baking sheet with cooking spray.
2. Halve the spaghetti squash, remove and discard the seeds, and place the halves cut-side down on the prepared baking sheet. Bake for 30 to 45 minutes, or until the flesh is tender and can be scraped with a fork.
3. Remove from the oven, and let cool. Scrape out the flesh with a fork, creating small noodles. Set aside.
4. In a small bowl, whisk together the soy sauce, garlic, oyster sauce, and ginger.
5. In a large skillet over medium heat, heat the oil. Add the onion and celery and cook, stirring, until tender, 3 to 4 minutes. Add the cabbage and cook, stirring, until heated through, 1 to 2 minutes.
6. Add the spaghetti squash and sauce mixture. Continue cooking for another 2 minutes.
7. Serve immediately.

Nutrition:
- Calories: 252
- Carbohydrates: 39 g
- Protein: 6 g
- Fat: 11 g
- Sodium: 950 mg

148. Zucchini Lasagna Roll-Ups

Preparation Time: 30 minutes
Cooking Time: 15 minutes
Servings: 1
Ingredients:

- 3 large zucchinis, trimmed and sliced lengthwise into -inch-thick strips
- 1 teaspoon salt
- Nonstick cooking spray
- 1 (10-ounce) bag fresh spinach
- 1 cup part-skim ricotta
- ½ cup Parmesan cheese
- 1 large egg
- 2 garlic cloves, minced
- 2 teaspoons Italian seasoning
- 1½ cups marinara sauce, divided
- 1 cup part-skim shredded mozzarella

Directions:

1. Preheat the oven to 400°F.
2. Lay the zucchini slices flat on a paper towel-lined baking sheet, and sprinkle with salt. Let sit for 15 minutes.
3. Meanwhile, spray a small skillet with nonstick cooking spray, and set over medium heat.
4. Add the spinach and cook for 2 minutes, or until wilted. Remove from the heat.
5. In a medium bowl, mix the ricotta, Parmesan, egg, garlic, and Italian seasoning until well combined.
6. Pat the zucchini dry, removing excess salt.
7. Spread 1 cup of marinara in the bottom of a 9-by-9-inch baking dish.
8. Spread each zucchini slice with a spoonful of ricotta mixture, then gently roll up and place in the prepared baking dish, seam-side down. Repeat with the remaining zucchini and filling.
9. Top with the remaining ½ cup of marinara, and sprinkle with the mozzarella cheese.
10. Bake for 25 to 30 minutes, or until the lasagna rolls are heated through and the cheese begins to brown.
11. Serve immediately.

Nutrition:
- Calories: 240
- Carbohydrates: 16 g
- Protein: 18 g
- Fat: 13 g
- Sodium: 1019 mg

149. Roasted Vegetable Quinoa Salad with Chickpeas

Preparation Time: 15 minutes
Cooking Time: 15 minutes
Servings: 1
Ingredients:

- 1 small eggplant, diced
- 1 small zucchini, diced
- 1 small yellow summer squash, diced
- ½ cup grape tomatoes, halved
- 1 (15-ounce) can chickpeas, drained and rinsed
- 3 tbsps. extra-virgin olive oil, divided
- 1/3 cup packaged quinoa
- 1 cup low-sodium vegetable or chicken broth
- 2 tbsps. freshly squeezed lemon juice
- 1 teaspoon minced fresh garlic or 1 garlic clove, minced
- 1 tbsp. dried basil
- 1 teaspoon dried oregano

Directions:

1. Preheat the oven to 425°F. Line a 9-by-13-inch baking sheet with parchment paper.

2. Spread the eggplant, zucchini, yellow squash, tomatoes, and chickpeas across the baking sheet and toss them with 1 tablespoon of olive oil.
3. Bake for 30 minutes, stirring once halfway through. The finished vegetables should be tender and the tomatoes should be juicy. The chickpeas will be firm and crispy.
4. While the vegetables and chickpeas are roasting, place the quinoa and broth in a small saucepan over medium-high heat. Cover and bring to a boil. Reduce the heat to low and cook for about 15 minutes, or until all liquid has absorbed. Remove the pan from the heat and fluff the quinoa with a fork. (Otherwise, make the quinoa according to the package instructions.)
5. In a small dish, whisk together the lemon juice, garlic, and the remaining 2 tablespoons of olive oil. Mix in the basil and oregano.
6. In a large serving bowl, combine the quinoa, roasted vegetables with chickpeas, and dressing. Gently stir to combine. Serve and enjoy!

Nutrition:
- Calories: 200
- Carbohydrates: 27 g
- Protein: 7 g
- Fat: 9 g
- Sodium: 160 mg

150. Mexican Stuffed Summer Squash

Preparation Time: 5 minutes
Cooking Time: 33 minutes
Servings: 1
Ingredients:
- Nonstick cooking spray
- 1 yellow summer squash
- ½ cup Refried Black Beans or canned fat-free refried pinto beans with 1 teaspoon taco seasoning mixed in (for flavor)
- ½ cup cooked quinoa
- ¼ cup shredded Colby Jack cheese
- 1 small tomato, diced
- 2 tbsps. sliced black olives
- 2 scallions, chopped, for garnish

Directions:
1. Preheat the oven to 400°F. Coat an 8-by-8-inch baking dish with the cooking spray.
2. Cut the ends off of the summer squash and discard. Cut lengthwise, then use a spoon to remove and discard the seeds. Place the squash halves cut-side down in the baking dish.
3. Gently poke a couple of holes in the squash to vent. Add 1 tablespoon of water to the dish. Microwave for about 3 minutes or until slightly tender. Discard any leftover water.
4. When cool enough to handle, turn the squash so they are skin-side down and spaced evenly apart in the dish.
5. Layer ¼ cup of the beans in each squash, then ¼ cup of the quinoa. Top the whole thing with the Colby Jack cheese. Cover with aluminum foil and bake for 25 minutes.
6. Remove the foil and bake for 5 minutes more, or until the cheese is bubbly and the squash is tender.
7. Garnish each squash with the tomatoes, olives, and scallions just before serving.

Nutrition:
- Calories: 190 Carbohydrates: 21 g
- Protein: 9 g
- Fat: 8 g
- Sodium: 40 mg

151. Tomato Bruschetta

Preparation Time: 15 minutes
Cooking Time: 5 minutes
Servings: 1
Ingredients:
- ½ finely chopped small red onion
- 8 medium coarsely chopped and drained tomatoes (about 500g)
- 2-3 crushed garlic cloves
- 6-8 leaves of finely chopped fresh basil
- 30 ml balsamic vinegar
- 60-80 ml extra virgin olive oil
- 1 crusty loaf of bread

Directions:
1. Mix the onions, tomatoes, garlic, and basil in a big bowl, taking care not to crush or break the tomatoes up too much. Balsamic vinegar and extra virgin olive oil should be added. As need, add salt and pepper. Again, combination. For at least an hour, cover and relax. This will make it easier to soak and mix the flavors.
2. Slice the baguette loaf into 12 thick slices diagonally and lightly toast them until both sides are light brown. On the warm bread slices, serve the mixture.

3. Take out from the freeze half an hour before serving if you like the mix at room temperature.

Nutrition:
- Calories: 310
- Carbohydrates: 42 g
- Protein: 8 g
- Fat: 12 g
- Sodium: 72 mg

152. Roasted Garlic Zucchini and Tomatoes

Preparation Time: 15 minutes
Cooking Time: 9 minutes
Servings: 1
Ingredients:
- 2 zucchinis cut in half lengthwise, then cut into 1/2-inch half-moons
- 2 cups quartered ripe tomatoes
- ½ onion, minced
- 3 cloves garlic, minced
- ½ tsp. crushed red pepper flakes
- ¼ cup of olive oil
- salt and pepper as needed
- ½ cup of grated Parmesan cheese
- 1 tbsp. chopped fresh basil

Directions:
1. Heat the oven to 450°F. Lightly grease a baking dish measuring 9x13 inches.
2. In the prepared baking dish, combine the zucchini, tomatoes, onion, garlic, and red pepper flakes. Add the olive oil and sprinkle, season with salt and pepper, and blend well.
3. Set in a preheated oven. Roast for about 18 minutes, until the vegetables are tender and slightly golden. Remove from the oven sprinkle with basil and Parmesan cheese.

Nutrition:
- Calories: 204
- Carbohydrates: 9.5 g
- Protein: 5.9 g
- Fat: 16.8 g
- Sodium: 165.2 mg

153. Soba Noodle & Edamame Salad with Grilled Tofu

Preparation Time: 15 minutes
Cooking Time: 8 minutes
Servings: 1
Ingredients:
- 140 g soba noodles
- 300 g fresh or frozen podded edamame (soy) beans
- 4 spring onions, shredded
- 300 g bag beansprouts
- 1 cucumber, peeled, halved lengthways, deseeded with a tsp. and sliced
- 250 g block firm tofu, patted dry and thickly sliced
- 1 tsp. oil
- a handful of coriander leaves, to serve

For the dressing:
- 3 tbsp. mirin
- 2 tsp. tamari
- 2 tbsp. orange juice
- 1 red chili, deseeded, if you like, and finely chopped

Directions:
1. In your smallest saucepan, heat the dressing ingredients, boil for 30 secs, and then set aside.
2. Boil noodles according to the instructions for the box, adding the edamame beans for the final cooking time of 2 mins. Rinse thoroughly under freezing water, drain thoroughly, and pour the spring onions, beansprouts, cucumbers, sesame oil, and warm dressing into a large bowl. If you like, season.
3. For 2-3 mins per hand, brush tofu with the veg oil, season, and griddle or grill-the tofu is very delicate, so turn carefully. Cover, the tofu salad, scatter with cilantro, and serve

Nutrition:
- Calories: 331
- Carbohydrates: 48 g
- Protein: 21 g
- Fat: 7 g
- Sodium: 1240 mg

154. Broccoli Casserole

Preparation Time: 1 minute
Cooking Time: 10 minutes
Servings: 1
Ingredients:
- 4 cups cut up broccoli
- As needed Ritz crackers
- 2 cups cheddar cheese

Directions:
1. Add the casserole ingredients into a Pyrex dish with the crumbled crackers on top.

2. Bake long enough to melt the cheese at 375°F.

Nutrition:
- Calories: 90.5
- Carbohydrates: 9.8 g
- Protein: 10.3 g
- Fat: 2.3 g

155. Chickpea and Feta Salad
Preparation Time: 7 minutes
Cooking Time: 0 minutes
Servings: 1
Ingredients:
- ¾ cup chopped raw vegetables
- ¼ cup each:
- 1 Can/fresh chickpeas
- Crumbled feta cheese
- 2 tablespoon lemon juice
- 2 tablespoons olive oil
- 1 teaspoon dried oregano
- Dash each of: pepper, salt

Directions:
1. Use your imagination for the chopped veggies. Include peppers, avocado, tomatoes, onions, and celery, or your favorites.
2. Rinse and drain the chickpeas.
3. Combine all of the ingredients and chill in the fridge until ready to serve.

Nutrition:
- Calories: 285.2 Carbohydrates: 22.2 g
- Protein: 10.2 g
- Fat: 18.4 g

156. Eggplant Pesto Mini Pizza
Preparation Time: 10 minutes
Cooking Time: 45 minutes
Servings: 1
Ingredients:
- Each chopped: 1 bell pepper, 1 tomato, 1 eggplant, 1 medium sliced red onion
- 1/8 teaspoon salt
- 2 cloves of garlic
- Pinch of oregano
- ¼ cup each: extra-virgin olive oil, pesto sauce, hummus, vegan parmesan cheese
- Sandwich thins – Arnold Orowheat
- Optional: pepper flakes

Directions:
1. Set the oven to 400°F.
2. Chop the vegetables and combine the oil, pepper, salt, oregano, and pepper flakes if desired. Arrange on a baking tin and toast for approximately 30 to 45 minutes or until they are done the way you like them.
3. Toast the buns and spread the hummus on them, add the veggies, and a bit of pesto sauce. Sprinkle with the vegan cheese and enjoy.

Nutrition:
- Calories: 405
- Carbohydrates: 40.6 g
- Protein: 11.4 g
- Fat: 24.5 g

157. Lentil Vegetarian Loaf
Preparation Time: 5 minutes
Cooking Time: 1 hour 30 minutes
Servings: 1
Ingredients:
- ½ cup rinsed – dried lentils
- 2 yellow onions
- 2 cups cooked brown rice
- 2 tablespoons canola/olive oil
- ½ cup ketchup
- 1 can tomato paste (6 ounces)
- 1 teaspoon each of: marjoram, garlic powder, sage, ½ cup - quartered cherry tomatoes, ¾ cup tomato/pasta sauce
- To taste: salt, more ketchup

Directions:
1. Preheat the oven to 350°F.
2. Rinse and cook the lentils in 3 to 4 cups of water for approximately 30 minutes.
3. Drain and slightly mash the lentils.
4. Peel and chop the onions. Cook in the oil until golden.
5. Combine the onions, lentils, tomato paste, rice, tomatoes, sauce, and spices into a large pot. Mix well.
6. Press the mixture into a well-greased baking dish with ½ cup of ketchup over the top.
7. Bake for one hour.

Nutrition:
- Calories: 254.2
- Carbohydrates: 44.9 g
- Protein: 10.9 g
- Fat: 4.4 g

158. Spinach Lasagna

Preparation Time: 10 minutes
Cooking Time: 45 minutes
Servings: 1
Ingredients:

- 1 large egg
- 2 cups cottage cheese (1% milk fat)
- 2 cups part-skim mozzarella cheese
- 10 oz baby spinach
- 1 jar spaghetti/marinara tomato sauce
- 1 cup water
- 9 lasagna noodles
- 1/8 teaspoon black pepper

Directions:

1. Program the oven temperature to 350°F.
2. Combine the thawed, drained spinach, one cup of mozzarella, cottage cheese, egg, and the seasonings in a large mixing bowl.
3. Spray a 9x13x2-inch casserole dish with some cooking spray.
4. Layer ½ cup of the sauce, 3 noodles, and ½ of the cheese mixture. Repeat, and top with the noodles one cup of mozzarella. Pour water around the edges and toothpicks on top to place a piece of foil over the noodles.
5. Bake covered for one hour to 1 ½ hour. Let it rest for 15 minutes.

Nutrition:

- Calories: 316.8
- Carbohydrates: 24.3 g
- Protein: 26.4 g
- Fat: 12.6 g

159. Vegetarian Frittata

Preparation Time: 15 minutes
Cooking Time: 30-35 minutes
Servings: 1
Ingredients:

- 6 oz button mushrooms
- 1 pound asparagus
- 1 shallot
- 1 garlic clove
- 1 tablespoon olive oil
- 1 small zucchini
- 6 large eggs
- 1/3 cup 1% milk
- ¼ teaspoon of freshly ground black pepper
- 1 teaspoon salt
- 1 tablespoon chopped chives
- Dash of nutmeg
- medium/1 large tomato
- ¼ cup freshly grated parmesan cheese

Directions:

1. Set the oven temperature to 350°F.
2. Prepare the Asparagus: Wash and trim cutting it into one-inch pieces. Blanche cut asparagus for one to two minutes. Shock it by adding it to ice water. Drain and set to the side.
3. Wash and slice the mushrooms. Sauté them in the oil for ten minutes using medium heat. Mince the shallots and garlic and add – cooking two more minutes. Transfer the mushrooms to a plate and set it aside.
4. Slice the zucchini lengthwise and into half-moon shapes.
5. Whisk the eggs, milk, chives, pepper, salt, and nutmeg in a large mixing dish. Add the mushroom mixture, asparagus, and zucchini.
6. Spray a two-quart baking dish with cooking spray and add the egg/veggie mixture.
7. Arrange the thinly sliced tomatoes on top and sprinkle it with the parmesan cheese.
8. Bake 30-35 minutes. You can place the frittata under the broiler for two to three minutes to brown the top.
9. Cool and serve at room temperature or straight from the fridge.

Nutrition:

- Calories: 146.2
- Carbohydrates: 7.4 g
- Protein: 10.6 g
- Fat: 8.8 g

160. Seitan Bites

Preparation Time: 15 minutes
Cooking Time: 15 minutes
Servings: 1
Ingredients:

- Nonstick cooking spray
- 1 large egg
- ½ cup flaxseed meal
- 1½ tbsps. garlic powder
- 1½ tbsps. onion powder
- 1 (8-ounce / 227-g) package seitan, cut into strips or small, 2-inch pieces
- ½ cup buffalo wing sauce

Directions:
1. Preheat the oven to 350°F (180°C). Coat a baking sheet with cooking spray.
2. In a medium bowl, whisk the egg.
3. In another medium bowl, mix together the flaxseed meal, garlic powder, and onion powder.
4. One by one, coat each seitan piece in egg, allowing the excess egg to drip off, then lightly coat with the dry mixture.
5. Gently transfer coated pieces to the prepared baking sheet. Bake for 12 to 15 minutes, or until crispy, flipping halfway through.
6. Transfer to a large bowl, and coat with the buffalo wing sauce.
7. Serve immediately.

Nutrition:
- Calories: 87
- Carbohydrates: 5 g
- Protein: 8 g
- Fat: 4 g
- Sugars: 0 g
- Fiber: 2 g
- Sodium: 517 mg

CHAPTER 11:

Seafood Recipes

161. Grilled Sardines

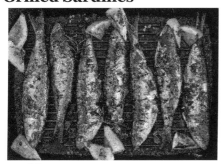

Preparation Time: 5 minutes
Cooking Time: 20 minutes
Servings: 4
Ingredients:

- 5 sardines
- Herbs of Provence

Directions:

1. Preheat the Air Fryer to 160°C.
2. Spray the basket and place your sardines in the basket of your fryer.
3. Set the timer for 14 minutes. After 7 minutes, remember to turn the sardines so that they are roasted on both sides.

Nutrition:

- Calories: 189g Fat: 10g
- Carbohydrates: 0g Sugars 0g
- Protein: 22g

162. Crunchy Air Fryer Fish

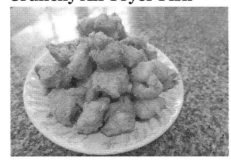

Preparation Time: 5 minutes
Cooking Time: 10/15 minutes
Servings: 4
Ingredients:

- 1/2 cup yellow cornmeal
- 1/2 tsp garlic powder
- 1 large egg
- 1 tsp coarse salt
- 1/2 tsp black pepper
- 1 lb. white fish fillets
- Lemon and parsley for garnish (Optional)
- Oil spray

Directions:

1. Preheat the Air Fryer for 3 minutes at 400°F.
2. Beat the egg in a shallow skillet.
3. In a different deep skillet, mix the cornmeal and spices.
4. Dry the fish completely.
5. Drop the fish fillets in the egg allow extra drip into the pan.
6. Press the fish into the cornmeal combination until well-crusted on the two sides.
7. Place the coated fish in the basket of the preheated fryer. Spray lightly with oil.
8. Cook for 10 minutes at 400°F, tossing the fish to ensure uniform cooking.
9. If there are dry spots, spray a little oil. Take back the basket to the Air Fryer and cook until the fish is well prepared.
10. Lightly squeeze with lemon and sprinkle with parsley.
11. Serve immediately.

Nutrition:

- Calories: 191
- Carbohydrates: 15 g
- Protein: 64 g
- Fat: 3 g

163. Tuna Zucchini Melts

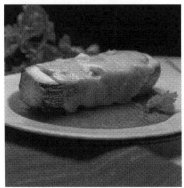

Preparation Time: 15 minutes
Cooking Time: 7/8 minutes
Servings: 4
Ingredients:

- 4 corn tortillas (unsalted)
- 3 tablespoons softened margarine
- 1 (6-ounce) can chunk light tuna, drained
- 1 cup shredded zucchini, drained by squeezing in a kitchen towel
- 1/3 cup mayonnaise
- 2 tablespoons mustard
- 1 cup parmesan cheese

Directions:

1. Coat tortillas with softened margarine.
2. Put in the basket of the Air Fryer and grill for 2 to 3 minutes at 350°F or until the tortillas are crispy
3. Take out of the basket and set aside.
4. Combine the tuna, zucchini, mayonnaise, and mustard in a medium bowl and mix well.
5. Split the tuna mixture between the toasted tortillas. Fold the tortillas together and top each tortilla with a little cheese.
6. Grill for 2-4 minutes in the Air Fryer at 350°F or until the tuna mixture is hot and cheese is melted and beginning to brown. Serve.

Nutrition:

- Calories: 228
- Total Fat: 30 g
- Carbohydrates: 19 g
- Protein: 52 g

164. Buttery Cod

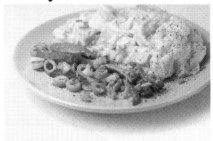

Preparation Time: 5 minutes
Cooking Time: 12/15 minutes
Servings: 4
Ingredients:

- 1 tbsp. parsley, chopped
- 3 tbsp. butter, melted
- 8 cherry tomatoes, halved
- ¼ cup tomato sauce
- 2 cod fillets, cubed

Directions:

1. Turn on the fryer to 390°F and heat for 2-3 minutes.
2. Combine butter, cherry tomatoes, tomato sauce, parsley, and cod fillets put them into a pan that works with the air fryer.
3. Place the pan in the Air Fryer and cook for about 12/15 minutes to 390°F.
4. After 12 minutes of cooking, divide into four bowls and enjoy.

Nutrition:

- Calories: 132
- Carbohydrates: 5 g
- Protein: 51 g
- Fat: 8 g

165. Breaded Coconut Shrimp

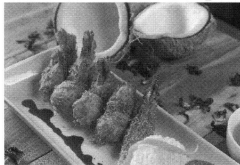

Preparation Time: 5 minutes
Cooking Time: 10/15 minutes
Servings: 4
Ingredients:

- 450 g shrimp
- 1 cup panko breadcrumbs

- 1 cup shredded coconut
- 2 eggs
- 1/3 cup all-purpose flour

Directions:
1. Preheat the Air Fryer to 360°Fahrenheit for 3-4 minutes.
2. Peel and devein the shrimp.
3. Pour the flour into a bowl.
4. In another bowl, beat the eggs, and in a third bowl, combine the breadcrumbs and coconut.
5. Dip the cleaned shrimp into the flour, eggs, and finish with the coconut mixture.
6. Lightly spray the fryer basket and bake for 10-15 minutes to 360°Fahrenheit or until golden brown.

Nutrition:
- Calories: 185
- Fat: 12.8 g
- Carbohydrates: 3.7 g
- Protein: 38.1 g

166. Codfish Nuggets

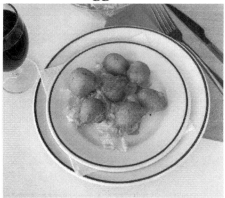

Preparation Time: 5 minutes
Cooking Time: 20 minutes
Servings: 4
Ingredients:
- 450 g Cod fillet
- 3 eggs
- 4 tbsp. olive oil
- 1 cup almond flour
- 1 cup gluten-free breadcrumbs
- Salt, to taste (very little)

Directions:
1. Heat the Air Fryer to 390°F.
2. Slice the cod into nuggets.
3. Prepare three bowls. Whisk the eggs in one. Combine the salt, oil, and breadcrumbs in another. Sift the almond flour into the third one.
4. Cover each of the nuggets with flour, dip in the eggs, and the breadcrumbs.
5. Arrange the nuggets in the basket and set the timer for 20 minutes and cook at 390°F.
6. Serve the fish with your favorite dips or sides.

Nutrition:
- Calories: 134
- Fat: 10 g
- Carbohydrates: 8 g
- Protein: 62 g

167. Easy Crab Sticks

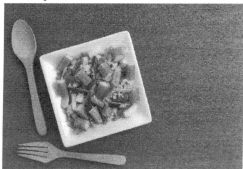

Preparation Time: 5 minutes
Cooking Time: 10 minutes
Servings: 4
Ingredients:
- 1 package Crab sticks
- Cooking oil spray, as needed

Directions:
1. Take each of the sticks out of the package and unroll it until the stick is flat.
2. Arrange them on the Air Fryer basket and lightly spritz using cooking spray. Set the timer for 10 minutes and cook at 385°F.
3. If you shred the crab meat, you can cut the time in half, but they will also easily fall through the holes in the basket.

Nutrition:
- Calories: 185
- Fat: 12.8 g
- Carbohydrates: 3.7 g
- Protein: 58.1 g

168. Fried Catfish

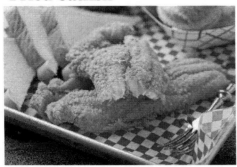

Preparation Time: 5 minutes
Cooking Time: 22/23 minutes
Servings: 4
Ingredients:

- 1 tbsp. olive oil
- 1/4 cup seasoned fish fry
- 4 Catfish fillets

Directions:

1. Heat the Air Fryer to reach 400°Fahrenheit before fry time. Rinse the catfish and pat dry using a paper towel.
2. Dump the seasoning into a sizeable zipper-type bag.
3. Add the fish and shake to cover each fillet. Spray with a spritz of cooking oil spray and add to the basket.
4. Set the timer for 10 minutes and cook at 400°Fahrenheit. Flip, and reset the timer for 10 additional minutes. Turn the fish once more and cook for 2-3 minutes.
5. Once it reaches the desired crispiness, transfer to a plate, and serve.

Nutrition:

- Calories: 176 Fat: 9 g
- Carbohydrates: 10 g Protein: 68 g

169. Zucchini with Tuna

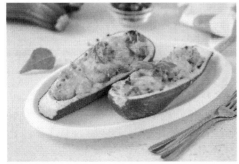

Preparation Time: 10 minutes
Cooking Time: 20/30 minutes
Servings: 4
Ingredients:

- 4 medium zucchinis
- 120 g of tuna in oil (canned) drained
- 30 g grated cheese
- 1 cup pine nuts
- Salt, pepper to taste (very little)

Directions:

1. Cut the zucchini in half laterally and empty it with a small spoon (set aside the pulp that will be used for filling)
2. Place zucchini in a Bowl.
3. In a food processor, put the zucchini pulp, drained tuna, pine nuts, and grated cheese. Mix everything until you get a homogeneous and dense mixture.
4. Fill the zucchini with the mixture.
5. Set the fryer to 180°CUP
6. Bake for 20/30 min. depending on the size of the zucchini. Allow cooling before serving

Nutrition:

- Calories: 139
- Carbohydrates: 10 g
- Fat: 29 g
- Protein: 53 g

170. Deep-Fried Prawns

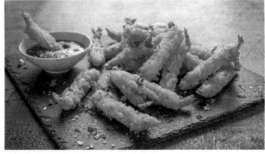

Preparation Time: 15 minutes
Cooking Time: 8/10 minutes
Servings: 6
Ingredients:

- 12 prawns
- 2 eggs
- Flour, to taste
- Breadcrumbs, to taste
- 1 tsp. oil

Directions:

1. Remove the head of the shrimp and carefully peel off the carapace.
2. In a bowl place the eggs and beat them, in another bowl the flour and in a third bowl the breadcrumbs.
3. Pass the prawns first in the flour, then in the beaten egg, and then in the breadcrumbs.
4. Preheat the Air Fryer for 1 minute at 150°C

5. Add the prawns and cook for 4 minutes. If the prawns are large, it will be necessary to cook 6 at a time.
6. Turn the prawns and cook for another 4 minutes.
7. They should be served with a yogurt or mayonnaise sauce.

Nutrition:
- Calories: 189
- Fat: 16
- Carbohydrates: 22.3 g
- Protein: 61.4 g

171. Monkfish with Olives and Capers

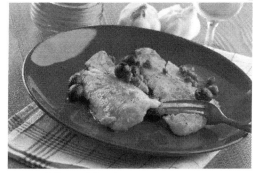

Preparation Time: 25 minutes
Cooking Time: 40 minutes
Servings: 4
Ingredients:
- 1 monkfish
- 10 cherry tomatoes
- 50 g olives
- 5 capers (unsalted)
- 1/2 tablespoons olive oil
- Salt, to taste (very little)

Directions:
1. Clean the monkfish well under running water and skin it completely using a sharp knife.
2. Lay a sheet of aluminum foil inside the basket of the Air Fryer and place the clean, skinless monkfish.
3. Add chopped tomatoes, olives, capers, oil, and salt.
4. Set the temperature of the Air Fryer to 160°C
5. Cook the monkfish for about 40 minutes or until we see the fish is cooked through and has become crispy.

Nutrition:
- Calories: 204 Fat: 19 g
- Carbohydrates: 26 g
- Protein: 54 g

172. Salmon with Pistachio Bark

Preparation Time: 10 minutes
Cooking Time: 25/30 minutes
Servings: 4
Ingredients:
- 600 g salmon fillet
- 50 g pistachios (unsalted)
- Salt to taste (very little)
- 1/2 tablespoons olive oil

Directions:
1. Put the parchment paper on the bottom of the Air Fryer basket and place the salmon fillet in it (it can be cooked whole or already divided into four portions).
2. Cut the pistachios into thick pieces, grease the top of the fish, salt (very little) and cover everything with the pistachios.
3. Set the fryer to 180°C and bake for 25/30 minutes.

Nutrition:
- Calories: 111.7
- Fat: 21.8 g
- Carbohydrates: 9.4 g
- Protein: 64.7 g

173. Easy Prawn Salad

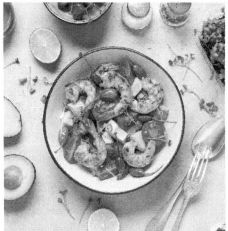

Preparation Time: 10 minutes
Cooking Time: 6/8 minutes
Servings: 4
Ingredients:
- 1/2 pounds king prawns, peeled and deveined
- Coarse sea salt and ground black pepper, to taste (very little)
- 1 tablespoon fresh lemon juice
- 1 cup mayonnaise
- 1 teaspoon Dijon mustard
- 1 tablespoon fresh parsley, roughly chopped
- 1 teaspoon fresh dill, minced

- 1 shallot, chopped
- Spray oil, to taste

Directions:
1. Toss the prawns with the salt and black pepper in a lightly greased Air Fryer cooking basket.
2. Cook the shrimp at 400°F for 6/8 minutes, shaking the basket halfway through cooking to turn the shrimp.
3. Add shrimp to a salad bowl add all remaining ingredients and mix well to season and blend everything together.

Nutrition:
- Calories: 241 Fat: 21.2 g
- Carbohydrates: 2.3 g Protein: 54.7 g

174. Fried Fish Fingers

Preparation Time: 10 minutes
Cooking Time: 10 minutes
Servings: 4
Ingredients:
- 2 eggs
- 1/42 cup all-purpose flour
- Sea salt and ground black pepper, to taste (very little)
- 1/2 teaspoon onion powder
- 1/4 teaspoon garlic powder
- 1/4 cup plain breadcrumbs
- 1/2 tablespoons olive oil
- 1 pound codfish fillets, slice into pieces

Directions:
1. In a bowl, place the eggs and beat with flour and spices.
2. In a separate bowl, thoroughly combine the breadcrumbs and olive oil.
3. Stir to combine the breadcrumbs with the oil well.
4. Now, dip the fish pieces into the flour mixture to coat them
5. Roll the fish pieces over the breadcrumb mixture until well coated on all sides.
6. Bake the fish sticks at 400°F for 10 minutes in the Air Fryer, turning them halfway through cooking.

Nutrition:
- Calories: 169
- Fat: 7.7 g
- Carbohydrates: 3.1 g
- Protein: 50.6 g

175. Salmon with Mushrooms and Bell Pepper

Preparation Time: 5 minutes
Cooking Time: 10 minutes
Servings: 2
Ingredients:
- ¼ cup oil
- ¼ cup flour, all-purpose
- 1 bell pepper
- 1 onion, chopped
- 1 lb. salmon fillet, sliced
- 4.5 oz mushrooms
- 2 tomatoes,
- 3 garlic cloves
- 1 tsp. soy sauce
- 1 1 tsp. sugar, white)
- Salt and pepper to taste
- 3 drops hot sauce

Directions:
1. Add oil into the Air Fryer pot.
2. Mix bell pepper, chicken, mushrooms, tomatoes, onion, soy sauce, garlic, sugar, and hot sauce.
3. Add salt and pepper with flour.
4. Cook at 300°F for 15 minutes.
5. When done, serve and enjoy!

Nutrition:
- Calories: 108
- Sodium: 52mg
- Protein: 110g
- Carbohydrates: 8g
- Fat: 10g
- Potassium: 877mg

176. Cod and Chicken Broth

Preparation Time: 6 minutes
Cooking Time: 5 minutes
Servings: 3
Ingredients:
- ½ cup butter
- 1 onion, chopped
- 1 pack broccoli, frozen
- 2 cans chicken broth
- 1 tbsp. garlic powder
- 1 lb. cod fillets, sliced
- 2/3 cup cornstarch
- 1 cup water

Directions:
1. Add butter and onion into the Air Fryer pot.

2. Mix cod, onion, cornstarch, water, garlic powder, broccoli, and chicken broth.
3. Cook at 300°F 15 minutes.
4. When ready, serve and enjoy!

Nutrition:
- Calories: 155
- Sodium: 775mg
- Protein: 40g
- Carbohydrates: 10g
- Fat: 7g
- Potassium: 209.8mg

177. Spinach with Tuna Fish

Preparation Time: 4 minutes
Cooking Time: 10 minutes
Servings: 2
Ingredients:
- 2 tbsp. butter
- 1 onion, chopped
- 2 garlic cloves
- 1 tbsp. cumin powder
- 1 tbsp. paprika
- 1 can tuna fish
- 2 tomatoes, chopped
- 2 cups vegetable broth
- 1 small bunch spinach, chopped
- Cilantro for garnishing

Directions:
1. Add butter into the Air Fryer pot.
2. Mix tuna fish, onion, garlic, cumin powder, paprika, and vegetable broth.
3. Add tomatoes and spinach.
4. Cook at 300°F for 10 minutes.
5. When ready, enjoy!

Nutrition:
- Calories: 95
- Sodium: 960mg
- Protein: 200g
- Carbohydrates: 10g
- Fat: 6g
- Potassium: 761mg

178. Sweet Potato with Tilapia

Preparation Time: 5 minutes
Cooking Time: 10 minutes
Servings: 2
Ingredients:
- 2 lbs. sweet potatoes, cubes
- 2 garlic cloves
- Salt to taste
- 1 lb. tilapia fillets
- 1 tbsp. sage
- 1 tbsp. rosemary
- 2 tbsp. butter
- 2 cups grated cheese

Directions:
1. Add garlic cloves into the Air Fryer pot.
2. Mix sage, butter, and rosemary.
3. Add sweet potatoes with salt.
4. Cook at 300°F for 10 minutes.
5. When ready, enjoy the tasty meal!

Nutrition:
- Calories: 90
- Sodium: 317mg
- Protein: 25g
- Carbohydrates: 20g
- Fat: 8g
- Potassium: 378mg

179. Kale with Tuna

Preparation Time: 4 minutes
Cooking Time: 10 minutes
Servings: 3
Ingredients:
- 12 cups kale, chopped–
- 2 tbsp. lemon juice
- 1 tbsp. oil
- 1 can tuna fish
- 1 tbsp. garlic, minced
- 1 tsp. soy sauce
- Salt and pepper to taste

Directions:
1. Add oil into the Air Fryer pot.
2. Mix tuna fish, garlic, soy sauce, lemon juice, kale, salt, and pepper.
3. Cook at 300°F for 10 minutes.
4. When ready, enjoy!

Nutrition:
- Calories: 90
- Sodium: 894mg
- Protein: 25g
- Carbohydrates: 20g
- Fat: 8g
- Potassium: 2170mg

180. Spinach with Salmon and Seashells

Preparation Time: 5 minutes
Cooking Time: 10 minutes
Servings: 3
Ingredients:
- 1 pound seashells

- 1 pack spinach, chopped
- 2 tbsp. oil
- 7 garlic cloves, minced
- 1 lb. salmon, chopped
- 1 tsp. red pepper flakes
- Salt to taste

Directions:
1. Add oil into the Air Fryer pot.
2. Mix tuna fish, garlic, red pepper flakes, spinach, and seashells with salt.
3. Cook at 300°F for 15 minutes.
4. When the pot beeps, serve and enjoy!

Nutrition:
- Calories: 100g Sodium: 440mg
- Protein: 110g Carbohydrates: 8g
- Fat: 10g Potassium: 0mg

181. Paprika Mix Salmon

Preparation Time: 6 minutes
Cooking Time: 8 minutes
Servings: 3
Ingredients:
- 1 onion, chopped
- 2 garlic cloves, chopped
- 1 carrot, chopped
- 2 stalks celery, sliced
- 1 tbsp. ginger root, minced
- ½ tsp. paprika
- ½ tsp. cumin powder
- ½ tsp. oregano
- 2 tomatoes, crushed
- 1 lb. salmon fillets
- 1 zucchini, sliced
- 1 tbsp lemon juice
- Salt to taste

Directions:
1. Add lemon juice into the Air Fryer pot.
2. Add onion, garlic, celery, ginger root, oregano, cumin powder, paprika, and carrots.
3. Add tomatoes and zucchini along with salt.
4. Cook at 300°F for 15 minutes.
5. When ready, serve and enjoy!

Nutrition:
- Calories: 95 Sodium: 937mg
- Protein: 200g Carbohydrates: 10g
- Fat: 6g
- Potassium: 740mg

182. Zucchini with Salmon Fillets

Preparation Time: 4 minutes
Cooking Time: 10 minutes
Servings: 2
Ingredients:
- 2 tbsp. canola oil
- 1 onion, chopped
- 1 zucchini, chopped
- 1 lb. salmon fillets
- 3 cups black beans
- 2 tomatoes, diced
- Salt and pepper to taste
- ½ cup corn
- Parsley to garnish

Directions:
1. Add oil into the Air Fryer pot.
2. Mix salmon fillets, onion, black beans, tomatoes, corn, zucchini, and salt and pepper.
3. Cook at 300°F for 10 minutes.
4. When done, garnish with parsley and serve.

Nutrition:
- Calories: 95 Sodium: 595mg
- Protein: 200g Carbohydrates: 10g
- Fat: 6g Potassium: 439mg

183. Black Beans with Ham and Salmon

Preparation Time: 4 minutes
Cooking Time: 9 minutes
Servings: 3
Ingredients:
- 2 lb. ham hock
- 1 lb. salmon, chopped
- 1 onion, chopped
- 2 garlic cloves, minced
- 2 cups black beans
- 2 bay leaves
- 2 tbsp. oregano powder

Directions:
1. Add onion and bay leaves into the Air Fryer pot.
2. Mix ham hock, garlic, black beans, and oregano powder.
3. Cook at 300°F for 9 minutes.
4. When done, serve and enjoy the meal!

Nutrition:
- Calories: 95 Sodium: 423mg
- Protein: 200g Carbohydrates: 10g
- Fat: 6g Potassium: 722mg

184. Tuna Fish with white Beans

Preparation Time: 6 minutes
Cooking Time: 10 minutes
Servings: 3
Ingredients:
- 1 tbsp. olive oil
- 2 tbsp. garlic, minced
- 2 cups spinach
- 2 tomatoes
- 3 cups white beans
- Salt and pepper to taste
- 1 can tuna fish
- Cheese to garnish

Directions:
1. Add oil into the Air Fryer pot.
2. Mix garlic and spinach.
3. Add tomatoes, white beans, and salt and pepper.
4. Cook at 300°F for 10 minutes.
5. When ready, garnish with cheese and serve!

Nutrition:
- Calories: 100 Sodium: 592mg
- Protein: 11g Carbohydrates: 8g
- Fat: 10g Potassium: 206mg

185. Kale and Salmon Fillets

Preparation Time: 5 minutes
Cooking Time: 8 minutes
Servings: 3
Ingredients:
- 2 tbsp. olive oil
- 2 tomatoes, chopped
- 2 potatoes, chopped
- Salt and pepper
- 2 cups kale, chopped
- 1 lb. salmon fillets

Directions:
1. Add oil into the Air Fryer pot.
2. Mix salmon fillets, potatoes, tomatoes, salt, and pepper with kale.
3. Cook at 300°F for 10 minutes.
4. When done, serve and enjoy!

Nutrition:
- Calories: 95
- Sodium: 340mg
- Protein: 200g
- Carbohydrates: 10g
- Fat: 6g
- Potassium: 0mg

186. Cod with Celery Stalk

Preparation Time: 6 minutes
Cooking Time: 10 minutes
Servings: 2
Ingredients:
- 2 carrots, sliced
- 2 cups vegetable broth
- 1 lb. Cod, cubed
- Salt to taste
- 4 cups cauliflower florets
- 2 tbsp. garlic, minced
- 2 tbsp. thyme, dried
- 4 celery stalks
- 1 tbsp. corn starch

Directions:
1. Add vegetable broth into the Air Fryer pot.
2. Add celery stalks, cornstarch, cod, thyme, garlic, cauliflower, salt, and carrots.
3. Cook at 300°F for 15 minutes.
4. When ready, serve and enjoy!

Nutrition:
- Calories: 90 Sodium: 607mg
- Protein: 25g Carbohydrates: 20g
- Fat: 8g Potassium: 1389mg

187. Squash with Salmon Fish

Preparation Time: 6 minutes
Cooking Time: 10 minutes
Servings: 3
Ingredients:
- 1 lb. squash
- 2 tbsp. butter
- 1 onion, chopped
- 2 garlic cloves, minced
- 3 cups chicken broth
- 2 tbsp. nutmeg powder
- Half and a half – ½ cup
- 1 lb. salmon fish, cubes

Directions:
1. Add butter into the Air Fryer pot.
2. Mix squash, chicken broth, salmon, garlic, onion, nutmeg powder, chicken breast, and a half and half. Cook at 300°F for 10 minutes. When done, serve and enjoy!

Nutrition:
- Calories: 100 Sodium: 716mg
- Protein: 110g Carbohydrates: 8g
- Fat: 10g Potassium: 1565mg

CHAPTER 12:

Snacks

188. Tacos Crispy Avocado

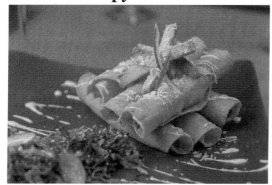

Preparation Time: 10 minutes
Cooking Time: 10 minutes
Servings: 5
Ingredients:
Salsa:

- 1 garlic clove, minced
- 1 Roma tomato, finely chopped
- 1 cup pineapple, finely chopped
- 1/2 red bell pepper, finely chopped
- 1/2 of a medium red onion
- Pinch each cumin and salt
- ½ not spicy jalapeno, finely chopped

Avocado tacos:

- 1 avocado
- 1/2 cup panko crumbs (65 g)
- 1 large egg whisked
- 1/4 cup all-purpose flour (35 g)
- 4 flour tortillas
- Pinch each salt and pepper

Adobo Sauce:

- 1/4 tsp lime juice
- 1/4 cup plain yogurt (60 g)
- 1 tbsp. Adobo sauce from a jar of chipotle peppers
- 2 tbsp. Mayonnaise (30 g)
- Polte peppers

Directions:

1. Sauce: mix all sauce ingredients together and refrigerate.
2. Prepare avocado: halve the length of the avocado, remove the stone and place the avocado skin face down cut each half into 4 equal pieces. Then gently peel off the skin.
3. Prep station: heat t Air Fryer to 190°C Arrange your work area so you have a bowl of flour, a bowl of whisked egg, a bowl of Panko with S & P, and a baking sheet lined with baking paper at the end.
4. Coating: dip each avocado slice in flour, egg, and then panko. Place on the prepared baking sheet and fry in the Air Fryer for 10 minutes at 190°C
5. Sauce: While cooking avocados, mix all sauce ingredients together.
6. Place salsa on a tortilla and add 2 pieces of avocado. Drizzle with salsa and serve immediately.

Nutrition:

- Calories: 93
- Protein: 53.7 g
- Fat: 13.25 g
- Carbohydrates: 4.69 g

189. Apple Chips With Cinnamon and Yogurt Sauce

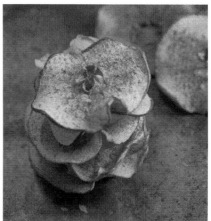

Preparation Time: 5 minutes
Cooking Time: 12 minutes
Servings: 4
Ingredients:

- 230 g apple (such as Fuji or Honeycrisp)

- 1 tsp. ground cinnamon
- 2 tsp. canola oil
- Cooking oil spray (as needed)
- 1/4 cup plain 1% low-fat Greek yogurt
- 1 tsp. honey
- 1 tbsp. almond butter

Directions:
1. Heat the fryer unit to reach 375°F/191°Celsius.
2. Thinly slice the apple on a mandoline. Toss the slices in a bowl with cinnamon and canola oil to evenly cover.
3. Spritz the fryer basket using cooking spray.
4. Arrange seven to eight sliced apples in the basket (single-layered).
5. Air-fry them for 12 minutes at 375°F (flipping them every 4 min.), and rearrange slices to flatten them. They will continue to crisp upon cooling. Continue the procedure with the rest of the apple slices.
6. Whisk the yogurt with the almond butter and honey in a mixing container until smooth.
7. Arrange six to eight sliced apples on each plate with a small dollop of dipping sauce.

Nutrition:
- Carbohydrates: 17 g Fat: 3 g
- Protein: 58 g
- Calories: 104

190. Mozzarella Cheese Bites with Marinara Sauce

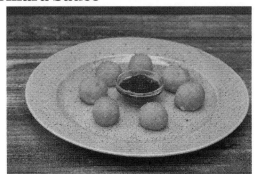

Preparation Time: 15 minutes
Cooking Time: 1 hour + 6/10 minutes
Servings: 12 cheese bites or 6 servings
Ingredients:
- 1 egg, lightly beaten
- 1 tbsp. water
- 1/2 cup all-purpose flour
- 1/2 tbsp. salt
- 1/2 tsp. dried Italian seasoning
- 3/4 cup panko breadcrumbs
- 6 Mozzarella cheese sticks
- Cooking spray
- 3/4 cup marinara sauce
- Red Pepper, to taste (very little)

Directions:
1. Slice the mozzarella cheese sticks in half—crosswise.
2. Whisk egg with water in a shallow mixing dish.
3. Stir the flour with salt and Italian seasoning in another shallow dish.
4. Place breadcrumbs in a third shallow dish.
5. Dip the cheese sticks into the egg mixture, then cover using the flour mixture. Dredge again into the egg mix, then into breadcrumbs until coated.
6. Arrange them on a baking tray—freeze until firm (1 hr.).
7. Preheat the Air Fryer to reach 360°Fahrenheit/182°Celsius.
8. Lightly coat the fryer basket using a spritz of cooking spray.
9. Place frozen cheese bites in the Air Fryer (single-layered), working in batches if necessary, being careful not to crowd.
10. Cook in the preheated Air Fryer until golden brown and cheese just begins to melt (4-6 min.). Repeat with the rest of the bites.
11. Meanwhile, whisk the marinara sauce and red pepper to your liking.
12. Serve the bites with marinara sauce.

Nutrition:
- Carbohydrates: 22.6 g Fat Content: 6.7 g
- Protein: 50.9 g Calories: 122.9

191. Spanakopita Bites

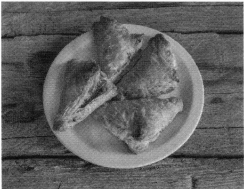

Preparation Time: 10 minutes
Cooking Time: 12 minutes
Servings: 8
Ingredients:
- 280 g baby spinach leaves

- 2 tbsp. water
- 1/4 cup 1% Low-fat cottage cheese
- 1/4 cup feta cheese, crumbled
- 2 tbsp. finely grated parmesan cheese
- 1 egg white
- 1 tsp. lemon zest
- 1/4 tsp each, black pepper and kosher salt
- 1/8 tsp. cayenne pepper
- 1 tsp. dried oregano
- 4 sheets frozen phyllo dough, thawed (13x18-inch/13x46-cm)
- 1 tbsp. olive oil
- Cooking spray

Directions:
1. Heat the Air Fryer to reach 375° Fahrenheit/191° Celsius.
2. Drain and add the spinach and water to a large pot. Simmer over high heat, stirring often until wilted (5 minutes).
3. Drain spinach and cool for about 10 minutes. Press firmly using some paper towels to remove as much moisture as possible.
4. Mix together the spinach, ricotta, feta, Parmesan, egg white, zest, oregano, salt, cayenne, and black pepper in a medium-sized bowl until well combined.
5. Place a sheet of phyllo on the work surface. Brush lightly with oil making use of a pastry brush. Top with the second sheet of phyllo and brush with oil.
6. Continue layering to form a stack of four oiled sheets. While working from the longer side, cut the stack of phyllo sheets into eight strips (21/4-inch wide). Slice the strips in half, crosswise, to form 16 strips 21/4 inches wide.
7. Pour about a tablespoon of filling onto one short end of each strip. Bend one corner over the filling to create a triangle - keep bending back and forth to the end of the strip, making a triangle-shaped phyllo package.
8. Lightly coat the fryer basket with cooking spray. Place eight packets seam-side down in the basket. Lightly spray the top. Cook until phyllo is nicely browned (12 min.), flipping packets halfway through the cooking process. Repeat with remaining phyllo packets

Nutrition:
- Carbohydrates: 27 g Fat: 4 g
- Protein: 64 g Calories: 82

192. Vegan-Friendly Kale Chips

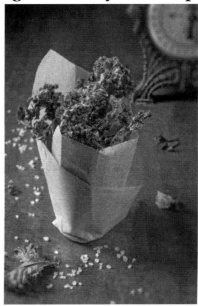

Preparation Time: 5 minutes
Cooking Time: 7 minutes
Servings: 2
Ingredients:
- 1 bunch curly kale
- 2 tsp. olive oil
- 1 tbsp. nutritional yeast
- 1/8 tsp. black pepper
- 1/4 tsp. sea salt

Directions:
1. Heat the Air Fryer unit to reach 390°Fahrenheit/199°Celsius.
2. Thoroughly rinse the kale and pat it dry. Remove the leaves from the stems of the kale and toss them into a mixing container.
3. Add the olive oil, salt, pepper, and nutritional yeast. Use your hands to massage the toppings into the kale leaves.
4. Scoop the kale into the basket of the fryer air-fry them until they are crispy (6-7 min.).
5. Note: If you are using a small Air Fryer, cook the chips in two batches. You don't want to overfill the fryer basket.
6. Enjoy them piping hot or slightly cooled.
7. Save any leftover chips in a zip-top bag for up to five days.

Nutrition:
- Carbohydrates: 9.1 g Fat: 5.3 g
- Protein: 33.8 g Calories: 90

193. Light Air-Fried Empanadas

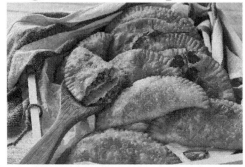

Preparation Time: 10 minutes
Cooking Time: 24 minutes
Servings: 2
Ingredients:

- 1 tbsp. olive oil
- 85 g 85/15 lean ground beef
- 1/4 cup white onion
- 85 g cremini mushrooms
- 2 tsp. garlic
- 6 pitted green olives
- 1/4 tsp. ground cumin
- 1/8 tsp. ground cinnamon
- 1/2 cup tomatoes
- 8 square gyoza wrappers
- 1 egg, lightly beaten

Directions:

1. Heat the Air Fryer unit to reach 400°Fahrenheit/204°Celsius.
2. Finely chop the onion, mushrooms, olives, and garlic. Also, chop the tomatoes or use canned.
3. Heat the oil in a skillet using the med-high temperature setting.
4. Add beef and onion to cook, stirring to crumble until brown (3 min.).
5. Mix in the mushrooms, occasionally stirring, until the mushrooms start to brown (6 min.).
6. Toss in the garlic, olives, cumin, and cinnamon cook until mushrooms are very tender and have released most of their liquid (3 min.).
7. Stir in tomatoes and cook for one minute, stirring intermittently.
8. Transfer the filling to a holding container and wait for it to cool (5 min.).
9. Arrange four wrappers on the work surface. Place about 1 1/2 tablespoons of filling in the middle of each wrapper. Brush each of the wrap's edges with egg and fold the wrappers over while pinching its edges to seal.
10. Repeat the process with the rest of the wrappers and filling.
11. Place four empanadas in the fryer basket (single-layered), and air-fry at 400°F them until nicely browned (7 min.).
12. Repeat with the remaining empanadas.

Nutrition:

- Carbohydrates: 25 g Fat: 19 g
- Protein: 57 g Calories: 182

194. Whole-Wheat Air-Fried Pizzas

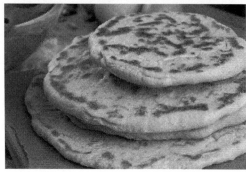

Preparation Time: 5 minutes
Cooking Time: 4/5 minutes
Servings: 2
Ingredients:

- 1/4 cup lower-sodium marinara sauce
- 2 whole-wheat pita rounds
- 1 cup baby spinach leaves
- 1 small plum tomato
- 1 small garlic clove
- 1/4 cup pre-shredded part-skim mozzarella cheese
- 1 tbsp. shaved Parmigiano-Reggiano cheese

Directions:

1. Heat the Air Fryer to 350°Fahrenheit/177°Celsius.
2. Spread the marinara sauce over one side of each pita bread.
3. Slice the tomato into eight slices and thinly slice the garlic.
4. Top each one-off using half of the spinach leaves, tomato slices, garlic, and cheeses.
5. Place one pita in the fryer basket, and air-fry to 350° F until the cheese is melted and the pita is crispy (4-5 min.).
6. Repeat with the remaining pita and serve.

Nutrition:

- Carbohydrates: 37 g
- Fat: 5 g
- Protein: 61 g
- Calories: 149

195. Zucchini Chips

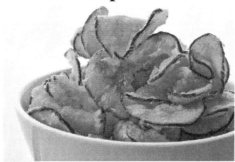

Preparation Time: 10 minutes
Cooking Time: 12/15 minutes
Servings: 5
Ingredients:

- 1.5 lb. zucchini
- 1/2 cup all-purpose flour
- 1 tsp. Italian seasoning
- 1/4 cup Parmesan/similar cheese, finely shredded
- Black pepper & salt, to taste (very little)
- 2 eggs
- 2 cups breadcrumbs
- Cooking oil spray, to taste

Directions:

1. Heat the Air Fryer unit to 400°Fahrenheit/204°Celsius.
2. Spritz the fryer basket with a tiny bit of cooking oil spray.
3. Break the eggs and add the flour and breadcrumbs into individual bowls.
4. Slice the zucchini into chips (1/4-inch thick). Use a mandolin for precise slicing to make the chips close to the same size for even cooking.
5. Whisk the flour with salt, pepper with a little shredded cheese.
6. Dip the zucchini pieces in the flour, egg, and lastly, the breadcrumbs before placing them in the fryer basket.
7. Spray the zucchini chips with cooking oil spray and air-fry for 5 minutes to 400°F.
8. Open the basket and flip the chips to spritz them with a tiny bit more oil.
9. Air-fry the zucchini chips until nicely browned (4-7 min.) to serve.

Nutrition:

- Carbohydrates: 31 g
- Fat: 4 g
- Protein: 69 g
- Calories: 107

196. Air-Fried Avocado Fries

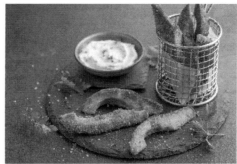

Preparation Time: 10 minutes
Cooking Time: 7-10 minutes
Servings: 2
Ingredients:

- 2 tbsp. all-purpose flour
- 1/8 tsp. salt
- 1/4 tsp. black pepper
- 1/2 egg
- 1/2 tsp. water
- 1/2 ripe avocado
- 1/4 cup panko breadcrumbs
- Cooking spray

Directions:

1. Preheat the Air Fryer unit to 400°Fahrenheit/204°Celsius.
2. Combine flour, pepper, and salt in a small shallow container.
3. Beat egg and water in a second shallow container. Place panko in a third shallow container.
4. Cut the avocado in half. Discard the seeds and peel.
5. Cut the prepared avocado into eight pieces.
6. Dip one slice of avocado in flour, patting off excess.
7. Dunk it in the egg and pat out the excess. Finally, press the slice into the panko so both sides are covered.
8. Place on a platter and replace with the remaining slices.
9. Generously spray the avocado slices with a cooking oil spray.
10. Place the slices in the Air Fryer bowl, spray side down. Also, spray the upper side of the avocado slices.
11. Cook in your pre-heated Air Fryer for 4 minutes to 400°Fahrenheit.
12. Flip the avocado slices and cook until golden brown (3 minutes).

Nutrition:

- Carbohydrates: 29.8 g Fat: 18 g
- Protein: 69.3 g Calories: 179

197. Chicken Nachos with Pepper

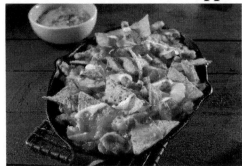

Preparation Time: 10 minutes
Cooking Time: 7/8 minutes
Servings: 6
Ingredients:

- 1 tbsp bean stew powder
- 1 tsp ground cumin
- 1 tsp salt
- ½ tsp ground dark pepper
- 1 tsp garlic powder
- 1/2 tsp new cleaved cilantro
- 1 pound ground chicken
- 1-pound red chime peppers cut into strips (not spicy)
- 1 ½ cups ground cheddar

Directions:
1. Preheat your Air Fryer to 400°F.
2. Combine the flavors in a little bowl.
3. Add the turkey to an enormous skillet and cook until caramelized. Mix in the zest blend.
4. Spot the pepper strips in a softly lubed heating container and top with the cooked chicken and cheddar.
5. Place Air Fryer-safe pan inside and cook for 8 minutes at 400°F or until cheddar has melted and turned brown.

Nutrition:
- Calories: 162
- Total Fat: 12 g
- Total Carbohydrates: 8 g
- Protein: 67 g

198. Dark Chocolate and Cranberry Granola Bars

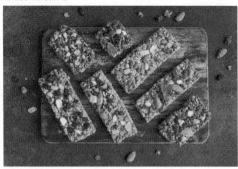

Preparation Time: 10 minutes
Cooking Time: 20 minutes
Servings: 8
Ingredients:

- 1 cup unsweetened shredded coconut
- 1 cup cut almonds
- ½ cup cleaved walnuts
- 1/3 cup dried cranberries
- 1/3 cup unsweetened, dim chocolate chips
- ½ cup hemp seeds
- ½ tsp salt
- ½ cup margarine
- 2 tsp keto maple syrup
- ½ cup powdered erythritol
- ½ tsp vanilla

Directions:
1. Preheat your Air Fryer to 300°F and line the Air Fryer plate with cooking paper.
2. Add the coconut, nuts, and hemp seeds to a food processor and pulse until very much blended and brittle.
3. Spot the blend in an enormous bowl alongside the cranberries, dull chocolate chips, and salt.
4. In a little pot, dissolve the margarine and maple syrup over low warmth.
5. Rush in the erythritol and mix until softened. Increase the heat and add the vanilla concentrate.
6. Pour the margarine blend over the nut blend and mix rapidly to cover uniformly.
7. Pour the blend onto the readied sheet plate and press down so the blend is leveled and even. Attempt to reduce it however much as could reasonably be expected so the bars hold together well.
8. Place the dish in the Air Fryer and bake for 20 minutes to 300°F. The edges should turn marginally brown.

9. Cool the bars totally and afterward cut and serve!

Nutrition:
- Calories: 149
- Total Fat: 12 g
- Total Carbohydrates: 6 g
- Protein: 63 g

199. Bacon Muffin Bites

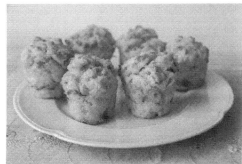

Preparation Time: 20 minutes
Cooking Time: 25 minutes
Servings: 24 little biscuits
Ingredients:
- 6 tbsp liquefied spread
- 1/4 cup minced garlic
- 1/2 cup acrid cream
- 4 eggs
- 2 cups almond flour
- 1 cup coconut flour
- 2 tsp preparing powder
- 1 cup destroyed cheddar
- ½ cup margarine
- 1/4 cup cleaved parsley
- 1/2 cup cooked, chopped bacon
- Salt, to taste (very little)

Directions:
1. Preheat your Air Fryer to 325°F and shower little biscuit tin or individual small-scale biscuit cups with cooking spray.
2. In a pan, over medium-high heat, cook the bacon, 5 to 7 minutes, flipping too evenly crisp. Dry out on paper towels, crumble, and set aside.
3. Spot the harsh cream, 1 tbsp garlic, eggs, and salt in a food processor, and puree until smooth.
4. Add the flours, cheddar, and parsley to the food processor and puree until a smooth mixture structure.
5. Overlap in the bacon chopped.
6. Melt the margarine
7. Distribute the mixture into the cookie cups.
8. Join the liquefied margarine and the leftover garlic and afterward brush the highest points of every biscuit with the spread blend.
9. Place the cookies in the deep fryer and bake for 18 minutes at 325°F or until the tops are bright earthy colored.
10. Cool before serving and appreciate!

Nutrition:
- Calories: 128
- Total Fat: 1 g
- Total Carbohydrates: 5 g
- Protein: 42 g

200. Brussels Sprout Chips

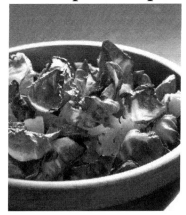

Preparation Time: 10 minutes
Cooking Time: 15 minutes
Servings: 4
Ingredients:
- 1 pound Brussels sprouts, closes eliminated
- 2 tbsp. olive oil
- 1 tsp ocean salt

Directions:
1. Preheat your Air Fryer to 240°F and line the Air Fryer plate with cooking paper.
2. Strip the Brussels sprouts each leaf in turn, setting the leaves in a huge bowl as you strip them.
3. Throw the leaves with olive oil and salt and afterward spread on the readied plate.
4. Place in the Air Fryer and cook for 15 minutes at 240°F, putting a little at a time to cook evenly.

Nutrition:
- Calories: 104
- Total Fat: 7 g
- Total Carbohydrates: 9 g
- Protein: 33 g

201. Herbed Parmesan Crackers

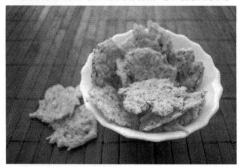

Preparation Time: 25 minutes
Cooking Time: 45 minutes
Servings: 10
Ingredients:

- 1 ½ cups sunflower seeds
- 3/4 cup parmesan cheddar, ground
- 2 tbsp Italian flavoring
- 1/2 cup chia seeds
- 1/2 tsp garlic powder
- 1/2 tsp heating powder
- 1 egg
- 2 tbsp. margarine, liquefied
- Salt, to taste (very little)

Directions:

1. Preheat your Air Fryer to 300°F.
2. Spot the sunflower seeds and chia seeds in a food processor until finely mixed into a powder. Spot in a huge bowl.
3. Add the cheddar, Italian flavoring, garlic powder, and preparing powder to the bowl and blend well.
4. Include the liquefied margarine and egg and mix until a pleasant mixture structure.
5. Spot the batter on a piece of cooking paper and afterward place another piece of cooking paper on top.
6. Fold the batter into a meager sheet around 1/8 inches thick.
7. Discard the top piece of paper towel and lift the batter using the base paper towel and place it on a plate that fits in the fryer.
8. Using the mixture, create the shape of crackers you want and place them in the Air Fryer to cook for 40-45 minutes at 300°F.
9. Split the saltines up and appreciate!

Nutrition:

- Calories: 173
- Total Fat: 18 g
- Total Carbohydrates: 9 g
- Protein: 39 g

202. Cauliflower Crunch

Preparation Time: 5 minutes
Cooking Time: 20/30 minutes
Servings: 4
Ingredients:

- 4 cups cauliflower florets, chopped into scaled-down pieces
- 1 tbsp olive oil
- 1 tsp ocean salt

Directions:

1. Preheat your Air Fryer to 135°F.
2. Wash and channel the cauliflower florets.
3. Spot the cauliflower in a big bowl and throw with the olive oil and ocean salt.
4. Add the cauliflower to the bushel of your Air Fryer or spread them in a level layer on the plate of your Air Fryer (either alternative will work!).
5. Cook in the Air Fryer for around 20/30 minutes to 135°F, turning the cauliflower consistently to cook uniformly. Basically, you will dry out the cauliflower.
6. When the cauliflower is completely dried, eliminate it from the Air Fryer and afterward let cool. It will stay fresh as it cools.
7. Appreciate fresh or store in an impenetrable compartment for as long as a month.

Nutrition:

- Calories: 55 Total Fat: 3 g
- Total Carbohydrates: 4 g
- Protein: 31 g

203. Lemon Pepper Broccoli Crunch

Preparation Time: 5 minutes
Cooking Time: 15/20 minutes
Servings: 4
Ingredients:

- 4 cups broccoli florets, slashed into reduced down pieces
- 1 tbsp olive oil
- 1 tsp ocean salt
- 1 tsp lemon pepper preparing

Directions:

1. Preheat your Air Fryer to 135°F.
2. Wash and channel the broccoli florets.
3. Spot the broccoli in an enormous bowl and throw it with the olive oil and ocean salt.
4. Add the broccoli to the container of your Air Fryer or spread them in a level layer on the plate of your Air Fryer (either choice will work!).

5. Cook in the Air Fryer for around 15/20 minutes to 135°F, turning the broccoli consistently to cook equitably. Basically, you will get dried out the broccoli.
6. When the broccoli is completely dried, take it out from the Air Fryer, throw with the lemon pepper preparing, and afterward let cool. It will stay fresh as it cools.
7. Appreciate fresh or store in a hermetically sealed compartment for as long as a month.

Nutrition:
- Calories: 53 Total Fat: 3 g
- Net Carbohydrates: 1 g
- Protein: 52 g

204. Delicate Garlic Parmesan Pretzels

Preparation Time: 15 minutes
Cooking Time: 12/14 minutes
Servings: 6
Ingredients:
- 2 cups almond flour
- 1 tbsp preparing powder
- 1 tsp garlic powder
- 1 tsp onion powder
- 3 eggs
- 5 tbsp mollified cream cheddar
- 3 cups mozzarella cheddar, ground
- 1 tsp ocean salt
- ½ tsp garlic powder
- ¼ cup parmesan cheddar

Directions:
1. Preheat your Air Fryer to 400°F and set up the Air Fryer plate with cooking paper.
2. Spot the almond flour, onion powder, preparing powder, and 1 tsp garlic powder in a big bowl and mix well.
3. Join the cream cheddar and mozzarella in a different bowl and dissolve in the microwave, warming gradually and mixing a few times to guarantee the cheddar liquefies and doesn't consume.
4. Add two eggs to the almond flour blend alongside the dissolved cheddar. Mix well until a mixture forms.
5. Separate the batter into six equivalent pieces and fold into your ideal pretzel shape.
6. Spot the pretzels on the readied sheet plate.
7. Whisk the excess eggs and brush over the pretzels, at that point sprinkle them all with the ocean salt, parmesan, and 1/2 tsp garlic powder. Cook in the Air Fryer for 12 minutes to 400°F or until the pretzels are brilliant earthy colored.
8. Remove from Air Fryer and appreciate it.

Nutrition:
- Calories: 193
- Total Fat: 39 g
- Total Carbohydrates: 10 g
- Protein: 48 g

205. Cucumber Chips

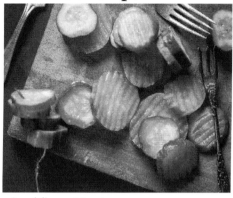

Preparation Time: 15 minutes
Cooking Time: 15 minutes
Servings: 4
Ingredients:
- 4 cups dainty cucumber cuts
- 2 tbsp apple juice vinegar
- 2 tsp ocean salt

Directions:
1. Preheat your Air Fryer to 200°F.
2. Spot the cucumber cuts on a paper towel and layer another paper towel on top to ingest the dampness in the cucumbers.
3. Spot the dried cuts in a huge bowl and throw with the vinegar and salt.
4. Place the cucumber cuts on a plate secured with paper towels and then cook in the fryer for 15 minutes to 200°F. The cucumbers will begin to twist and brown a bit.
5. Turn off the Air Fryer and let the cucumber cuts cool inside the fryer (this will help them dry somewhat more).
6. Appreciate immediately or store in an impermeable holder.

Nutrition:
- Calories: 15 Total Fat: 0 g
- Total Carbohydrates: 4 g
- Protein: 31 g

206. Cajun Cauliflower Crunch

Preparation Time: 5 minutes
Cooking Time: 15/20 minutes
Servings: 4
Ingredients:

- 4 cups cauliflower florets, chopped into scaled-down pieces
- 1 tbsp olive oil
- 1 tsp ocean salt
- 1 tsp Cajun preparing

Directions:

1. Preheat your Air Fryer to 135°F.
2. Wash and channel the cauliflower florets.
3. Spot the cauliflower in a huge bowl and throw with the olive oil and ocean salt.
4. Add the cauliflower to the crate of your Air Fryer or spread them in a level layer on the plate of your Air Fryer (either alternative will work!).
5. Place them in the Air Fryer to cook for about 15 to 20 minutes at 135°F, turning the cauliflower constantly to cook it evenly. Basically, you will dry out the cauliflower.
6. When the cauliflower is completely dried, eliminate it from the Air Fryer, throw with the Cajun preparing, and afterward let cool. It will stay fresh as it cools.
7. Appreciate fresh or store in a water/airproof holder for as long as a month.

Nutrition:

- Calories: 39 Total Fat: 3 g
- Total Carbohydrates: 4 g Protein: 41 g

207. Sprouts Wraps

Preparation Time: 5 minutes
Cooking Time: 20 minutes
Servings: 12
Ingredients:

- 12 bacon strips
- 12 Brussels sprouts A drizzle of olive oil

Directions:

1. Wrap each Brussels sprouts in a bacon strip, brush them with some oil, put them in your Air Fryer's basket, and cook at 350°F for 20 minutes. Serve as a snack.

Nutrition:

- Calories: 90
- Fat: 5 g
- Carbohydrates: 4 g
- Protein: 54 g

208. Pickled Bacon Bowls

Preparation Time: 5 minutes
Cooking Time: 20 minutes
Servings: 4
Ingredients:

- 4 dill pickle spears, sliced in half and quartered 8 bacon slices, halved
- 1 cup avocado mayonnaise

Directions:

1. Wrap each pickle spear in a bacon slice, put them in your Air Fryer's basket, and cook at 400°F for 20 minutes.
2. Divide into bowls and serve as a snack with mayonnaise.

Nutrition:

- Calories: 100 Fat: 4 g
- Carbohydrates: 3 g
- Protein: 54 g

209. Curried Brussels Sprouts

Preparation Time: 5 minutes
Cooking Time: 25 minutes
Servings: 1
Ingredients:

- 1 lb. Brussels Sprouts, ends trimmed & halved
- 2 teaspoons Olive Oil
- 1 tablespoon Lemon Juice, Fresh
- 3 teaspoons Curry Powder, Divided

Directions:

1. Start by getting gout in a large bowl and mix together your olive oil with a teaspoon of curry powder. Toss your Brussels sprouts in, mixing until well coated. Place them in your Air Fryer basket, roasting for twelve minutes. During this cooking time, you'll need to shake your basket once.
2. Sprinkle with the remaining curry powder and lemon juice, shaking your basket again. Roast for an additional three to five minutes. Your Brussels sprouts should be crisp and browned. Serve warm.

Nutrition:

- Calories: 86 Protein: 4 g
- Fat: 3 g Carbohydrates: 12 g

210. Crispy Cauliflower Bites

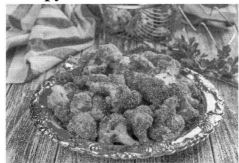

Preparation Time: 5 minutes
Cooking Time: 15 minutes
Servings: 1
Ingredients:

- 1 tbsp Italian seasoning
- 1 cup flour
- 1 cup milk
- 1 egg, beaten
- 1 head cauliflower, cut into florets

Directions:

1. Preheat Air Fryer to 390°F. Grease the Air Fryer basket with cooking spray. In a bowl, mix the flour, milk, egg, and Italian seasoning. Coat the cauliflower in the mixture and drain the excess liquid.
2. Place the florets in the frying basket, spray them with cooking spray, and Air Fry for 7 minutes. Shake and continue cooking for another 5 minutes. Allow cooling before serving.

Nutrition:

- Calories: 70 Carbohydrates: 2 g
- Fat: 1 g Protein: 3 g

211. Garlic Asparagus

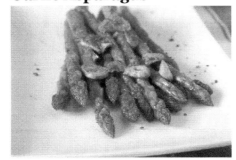

Preparation Time: 5 minutes
Cooking Time: 10 minutes
Servings: 1
Ingredients:

- 1 lb. asparagus, rinsed & trimmed
- 2 teaspoons olive oil
- 3 cloves garlic, minced
- 2 tablespoons balsamic vinegar
- ½ teaspoon thyme

Directions:

1. Start by getting out a large bowl to toss your asparagus in olive oil before placing your vegetables in the Air Fryer basket.
2. Sprinkle with garlic before roasting for eight to eleven minutes. Your asparagus should be tender but crisp.
3. Drizzle with thyme and balsamic vinegar before serving warm.

Nutrition:

- Calories: 41 Protein: 3 g
- Fat: 1 g Carbohydrates: 6 g

212. Crispy Kale Chips

Preparation Time: 5 minutes
Cooking Time: 10 minutes
Servings: 1
Ingredients:

- 4 cups kale leaves, stems removed, chopped
- 2 tbsp olive oil
- 1 tsp garlic powder
- Salt and black pepper to taste
- ¼ tsp onion powder

Directions:

1. In a bowl, mix kale and olive oil. Add in garlic and onion powders, salt, and black pepper toss to coat.
2. Arrange the kale in the frying basket and Air Fry for 8 minutes at 350°F, shaking once. Serve cool.

Nutrition:

- Calories: 80 Carbohydrates: 3 g
- Fat: 1 g Protein: 3 g

213. Crispy Squash

Preparation Time: 5 minutes
Cooking Time: 20 minutes
Servings: 1
Ingredients:

- 2 cups butternut squash, cubed
- 2 tbsp olive oil
- Salt and black pepper to taste
- ¼ tsp dried thyme
- 1 tbsp fresh parsley, finely chopped

Directions:

1. In a bowl, add squash, olive oil, salt, pepper, and thyme, and toss to coat.

2. Place the squash in the Air Fryer and Air Fry for 14 minutes at 360°F, shaking once or twice. Serve sprinkled with fresh parsley.

Nutrition:
- Calories: 100
- Carbohydrates: 5 g
- Fat: 2 g
- Protein: 3 g

214. Garlic Mozzarella Sticks

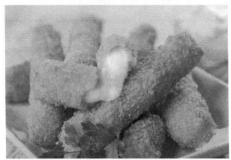

Preparation Time: 1 hour and 5 minutes
Cooking Time: 10 minutes
Servings: 1
Ingredients:
- 1 tablespoon Italian seasoning
- 1 cup parmesan cheese
- 8 strips cheese, cut into cubes
- 2 eggs, beaten
- 1 garlic clove, minced

Directions:
1. Start by combining your parmesan, garlic, and Italian seasoning in a bowl. Dip your cheese into the egg, and mix well.
2. Roll it into your cheese crumbles, and then press the crumbs into the cheese.
3. Place them in the fridge for an hour, and then preheat your Air Fryer to 375°F.
4. Spray your Air Fryer down with oil, and then arrange the cheese strings into the basket. Cook for eight to nine minutes at 365°F.
5. Allow them to cool for at least five minutes before serving.

Nutrition:
- Calories: 80 Protein: 7 g
- Fat: 6.2 g Net Carbohydrates: 3 g

215. Homemade Peanut Corn Nuts

Preparation Time: 5 minutes
Cooking Time: 20 minutes
Servings: 1
Ingredients:
- 6 oz dried hominy, soaked overnight
- 3 tbsp peanut oil
- 2 tbsp old bay seasoning
- Salt to taste

Directions:
1. Preheat Air Fryer to 390°F.
2. Pat dry hominy and season with salt and old bay seasoning. Drizzle with oil and toss to coat. Spread in the Air Fryer basket and Air Fry for 10-12 minutes. Remove to shake up and return to cook for 10 more minutes until crispy.
3. Transfer to a towel-lined plate to soak up the excess fat. Let cool and serve.

Nutrition:
- Calories: 100
- Carbohydrates: 3 g
- Fat: 3 g
- Protein: 5 g

216. Divided Balsamic Mustard Greens

Preparation Time: 17 minutes
Cooking Time: 15 minutes
Servings: 1
Ingredients:
- 1 bunch mustard greens, trimmed
- 2 tablespoons olive oil
- ½ cup chicken stock
- 2 tablespoons tomato puree
- 3 garlic cloves, minced
- Salt and black pepper to taste
- 1 tablespoon balsamic vinegar-

Directions:
1. Mix all of the ingredients in a pan that fits right into your Air Fryer and toss well.
2. Move the pan to the fryer and cook at a temperature of 260°F for 12 minutes.
3. Divide all of it into different plates, serve your meal, and enjoy!

Nutrition:
- Calories: 151 Fat: 2 g
- Fiber: 4 g
- Carbohydrates: 14 g
- Protein: 4 g

217. Honey Roasted Carrots

Preparation Time: 5 minutes
Cooking Time: 20 minutes
Servings: 1
Ingredients:
- 1 tablespoon honey, raw

- 3 cups baby carrots
- 1 tablespoon olive oil
- Sea salt & black pepper to taste

Directions:
1. Put all of the ingredients in a bowl, then heat your Air Fryer to 390°F.
2. Cook for 12 minutes and serve warm.

Nutrition:
- Calories: 82
- Protein: 1 g
- Fat: 3.2 g
- Carbohydrates: 2.1 g

218. Roasted Bell Pepper

Preparation Time: 5 minutes
Cooking Time: 20 minutes
Servings: 1
Ingredients:
- 1 teaspoon olive oil
- ½ teaspoon thyme
- 4 garlic cloves, minced
- 4 bell peppers, cut into fourths

Directions:
1. Start by putting your peppers in your Air Fryer basket and drizzling with olive oil. Make sure they're coated well and then roast for fifteen minutes.
2. Sprinkle with thyme and garlic, roasting for an additional three to five minutes. They should be tender and serve warm.

Nutrition:
- Calories: 36
- Protein: 1 g
- Fat: 1 g
- Carbohydrates: 5 g

219. Baked Potatoes with Bacon

Preparation Time: 5 minutes
Cooking Time: 30 minutes
Servings: 1
Ingredients:
- 4 potatoes, scrubbed, halved, cut lengthwise
- 1 tbsp. olive oil
- Salt and black pepper to taste
- 4 oz bacon, chopped

Directions:
1. Preheat the Air Fryer to 390°F. Brush the potatoes with olive oil and season with salt and pepper. Arrange them in the greased frying basket, cut-side down.
2. Bake for 15 minutes, flip them, top with bacon, and bake for 12-15 minutes or until potatoes are golden and bacon is crispy. Serve warm.

Nutrition:
- Calories: 150
- Carbohydrates: 9 g
- Fat: 7 g
- Protein: 12 g

220. Chicken Thighs

Preparation Time: 5 minutes
Cooking Time: 15 minutes
Servings: 1
Ingredients:
- 1 ½ lb. chicken thighs
- 2 eggs, lightly beaten
- 1 cup seasoned breadcrumbs
- ½ tsp oregano
- Salt and black pepper, to taste

Directions:
1. Preheat the Air Fryer to 390°F. Season the chicken with oregano, salt, and pepper. In a bowl, add the beaten eggs. In a separate bowl, add the breadcrumbs. Dip chicken thighs in the egg wash, then roll them in the breadcrumbs and press firmly so the breadcrumbs stick well.
2. Spray the chicken with cooking spray and arrange it on the frying basket in a single layer, skin-side up.
3. Air Fry for 12 minutes, turn the chicken thighs over, and continue cooking for 6-8 more minutes. Serve.

Nutrition:
- Calories: 190
- Carbohydrates: 11 g
- Fat: 8 g
- Protein: 16 g

221. Corn-Crusted Chicken Tenders

Preparation Time: 10 minutes
Cooking Time: 15 minutes
Servings: 1
Ingredients:
- 2 Chicken breasts, cut into strips
- Salt and black pepper to taste
- 2 eggs
- 1 cup ground cornmeal

Directions:
1. Preheat Air Fryer to 390°F.

2. In a bowl, mix ground cornmeal, salt, and black pepper. In another bowl, beat the eggs season with salt and pepper. Dip the chicken in the eggs and then coat in cornmeal. Spray the prepared sticks with cooking spray and place them in the Air Fryer basket in a single layer.
3. Air Fry for 6 minutes, slide the basket out and flip the sticks cook for 6-8 more minutes until golden brown.

Nutrition:
- Calories: 170
- Carbohydrates: 8 g
- Fat: 6 g
- Protein: 16 g

222. Simple Buttered Potatoes

Preparation Time: 5 minutes
Cooking Time: 30 minutes
Servings: 1
Ingredients:
- 1-pound potatoes, cut into wedges
- 2 garlic cloves, grated
- 1 tsp fennel seeds
- 2 tbsp butter, melted
- Salt and black pepper to taste

Directions:
1. In a bowl, mix the potatoes, butter, garlic, fennel seeds, salt, and black pepper, until they are well-coated. Set up the potatoes in the Air Fryer basket.
2. Bake at 360°F for 25 minutes, shaking once during cooking until crispy on the outside and tender on the inside. Serve warm.

Nutrition:
- Calories: 100
- Carbohydrates: 8 g
- Fat: 4 g
- Protein: 7 g

223. Roasted Coconut Carrots

Preparation Time: 5 minutes
Cooking Time: 10 minutes
Servings: 1
Ingredients:
- 1 tbsp coconut oil, melted
- 1 lb. horse carrots, sliced
- Salt and black pepper to taste
- ½ tsp chili powder

Directions:
1. Preheat Air Fryer to 400°F.
2. In a bowl, mix the carrots with coconut oil, chili powder, salt, and pepper. Place in the Air Fryer and Air Fry for 7 minutes.
3. Shake the basket and cook for another 5 minutes until golden brown. Serve.

Nutrition:
- Calories: 80
- Carbohydrates: 3 g
- Fat: 1 g
- Protein: 4 g

224. BBQ Chicken

Preparation Time: 5 minutes
Cooking Time: 30 minutes
Servings: 1
Ingredients:
- 1 whole small chicken, cut into pieces
- 1 tsp salt
- 1 tsp smoked paprika
- 1 tsp garlic powder
- 1 cup BBQ sauce

Directions:
1. Mix salt, paprika, and garlic powder and coat the chicken pieces. Place in the Air Fryer basket and bake for 18 minutes at 400°F. Remove to a plate and brush with barbecue sauce.
2. Wipe the fryer clean from the chicken fat. Return the chicken to the fryer, skin-side up, and bake for 5 more minutes at 340°F.

Nutrition:
- Calories: 230
- Carbohydrates: 12 g
- Fat: 9 g
- Protein: 23 g

225. Pork Rinds

Preparation Time: 5 minutes
Cooking Time: 10 minutes
Servings: 1
Ingredients:
- ½ teaspoon black pepper
- 1 teaspoon chili flakes
- ½ teaspoon sea salt, fine
- 1 teaspoon olive oil
- 1 lb. Pork rinds

Directions:
1. Start by heating your Air Fryer to 365°F, and then spray it down with olive oil.

2. Place your pork rinds in your Air Fryer basket, and sprinkle with your seasoning. Mix well, and then cook for seven minutes.
3. Shake gently, and then serve cooled.

Nutrition:
- Calories: 329 Protein: 36.5 g
- Fat: 20.8 g Net Carbohydrates: 0.1 g

226. Crispy Brussels Sprouts And Potatoes

Preparation Time: 10 minutes
Cooking Time: 8 minutes
Servings: 1
Ingredients:
- ¾ pound Brussels sprouts, washed and trimmed
- ½ cup new potatoes, chopped
- 2 teaspoons bread crumbs
- Salt and black pepper, to taste
- 2 teaspoons butter

Directions:
1. In a bowl, add Brussels sprouts, potatoes, bread crumbs, salt, pepper, and butter. Mix well.
2. Place in the Air Fryer and cook at 400°F for 8 minutes. Serve.

Nutrition:
- Calories: 152 Fat: 3g
- Carb: 17g Protein: 4g

227. Duck Fat Roasted Red Potatoes

Preparation Time: 5 minutes
Cooking Time: 25 minutes
Servings: 1
Ingredients:
- 4 red potatoes, cut into wedges
- 1 tbsp garlic powder
- Salt and black pepper to taste
- 2 tbsp thyme, chopped
- 3 tbsp duck fat, melted

Directions:
1. Preheat the Air Fryer to 380°F. In a bowl, mix duck fat, garlic powder, salt, and pepper. Add the potatoes and shake to coat.
2. Place in the basket and bake for 12 minutes, remove the basket, shake and continue cooking for another 8-10 minutes until golden brown. Serve warm topped with thyme.

Nutrition:
- Calories: 110 Carbohydrates: 8 g
- Fat: 5 g Protein: 7 g

CHAPTER 13:

Dessert Recipes

228. Chocolate Mug Cake

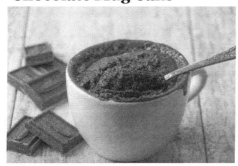

Preparation Time: 7 minutes
Cooking Time: 13 minutes
Servings: 3
Ingredients:

- ½ cup of cocoa powder
- ½ cup stevia powder
- 1 cup coconut cream
- 1 package cream cheese, room temperature
- 1 tbsp. vanilla extract
- 1 tbsp. butter

Directions:

1. Smart Air Fryer Oven is prepared at 350°F for a further 5 minutes.
2. Using a hand mixer, blend all the mentioned ingredients until frothy.
3. Put them into fatty cups.
4. In the fryer basket, place the cups and bake at 350°F for 13 minutes.
5. Serve as cold as possible.

Nutrition:

- Calories: 100
- Fat: 0 g
- Carbohydrates: 21 g
- Sugar 6 g
- Protein: 3 g

229. Chocolate Soufflé

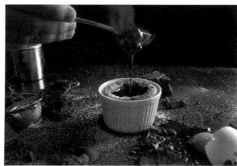

Preparation Time: 7 minutes
Cooking Time: 12 minutes
Servings: 2
Ingredients:

- 1 tbsp. Almond flour
- ½ tsp. vanilla
- 1 tbsp. sweetener
- 2 separated eggs
- ¼ cups melted coconut oil
- 4 oz. of semi-sweet chocolate, chopped

Directions:

1. Preheat the Smart Air Fryer Oven to 330°F.
2. Brush coconut oil and sweetener onto ramekins.
3. Melt coconut oil and chocolate together.
4. Beat egg yolks well, adding vanilla and sweetener.
5. Stir in flour and ensure there are no lumps.
6. Whisk egg whites till they reach peak state and fold them into chocolate mixture.
7. Pour batter into ramekins and place into the Smart Air Fryer Oven, then cook for 12 minutes.
8. Serve with powdered sugar dusted on top.

Nutrition:

- Calories: 612 Fat: 43g
- Carbohydrates: 46g Protein: 9g

230. Chocolate Cake

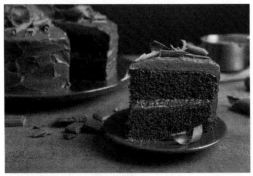

Preparation Time: 6 minutes
Cooking Time: 35 minutes
Servings: 9
Ingredients:

- ½ cups hot water
- 1 tsp. vanilla
- ¼ cups olive oil
- ½ cups almond milk
- 1 egg - ½ tsp. Salt
- ¾ tsp. baking soda
- ¾ tsp. baking powder
- ½ cups unsweetened cocoa powder
- 2 cups almond flour
- 1 cup brown sugar

Directions:

1. Turn the Smart Air Fryer Oven to 356°F.
2. Mix the dry ingredients and then stir in the wet.
3. Add hot water last.
4. The thin batter is better.
5. Bake a cake batter-sized pan in the fryer.
6. Bake for 35 minutes.

Nutrition:

- 214 calories Protein: 3.2g
- Carbohydrates: 25.5g Fat: 11.7g
- Cholesterol: 73.2mg Sodium: 130.3mg

231. Choc Chip Air Fryer Cookies

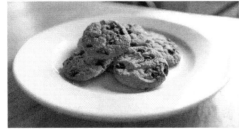

Preparation Time: 10 minutes
Cooking Time: 16 minutes
Servings: 3
Ingredients:

- 75 g self raising flour
- 100 g butter
- 75 g brown sugar
- 75 g milk chocolate
- 30 milliliters honey
- 30 milliliters whole milk

Directions:

1. Beat the butter until smooth and fluffy.
2. Add the butter to the sugar and beat together in a smooth mixture.
3. Now add and mix in the milk, sugar, chocolate (broken into small chunks/chips), and flour.
4. Preheat your Air Fryer to 360F.
5. Form the mixture into cookie shapes and place on a baking sheet that will rest in the Air Fryer for 16 minutes. Use (heat) the oven.

Nutrition:

- Calories: 179 Fat: 9g
- Carbohydrates: 22g Protein: 2g
- Cholesterol: 23 mg

232. Doughnuts

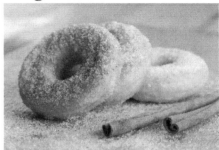

Preparation Time: 35 minutes
Cooking Time: 60 minutes
Servings: 8 (serving size: 1 doughnut)
Ingredients:

- 1/4 cup warm water, warmed (100°F to 110°F)
- 1 tablespoon active yeast
- 1/4 cup, plus half tsp. Granulated sugar, divided
- 2 cups (about 8 1/2 oz.) all-purpose flour
- 1/4 teaspoon kosher salt
- 1/4 cup of whole milk, at room temperature
- 2 tablespoons unsalted butter, melted
- 1 large egg, beaten
- 1 cup (about 4 oz.) powdered Sugar
- 4 teaspoons tap water

Directions:

1. Mix water, yeast, and 1/2 teaspoon of granulated sugar in a small bowl let rest for about five minutes. Combine flour, salt, and remaining 1/4-cup granulated sugar in a medium bowl.

2. Add yeast, milk, butter, and egg stir with a spoon until a soft dough is mixed. Switch to an oiled tub. Cover until doubled in volume, about 1 hour.
3. Turn dough onto a floured surface. Gently roll to 1/4-inch. To remove the core, cut eight doughnuts with a 3-inch round cutter and a 1-inch round cutter: place doughnuts and doughnuts on a lightly floured board. Cover plastic wrap loosely and let stand for about 30 minutes, until doubled in volume.
4. Place two doughnuts and two doughnuts in a single layer in an Air Fryer pan and cook 4 to 5 minutes at 350°F until golden brown. Continue with the rest of the doughnuts and holes.
5. Whisk powdered sugar together, tap water in a medium bowl until smooth. Place them in a glaze on a wire rack positioned atop a rimmed baking sheet to let excess glaze drop off. Let stand for 10 minutes until the glaze sets.

Nutrition:
- Calories: 342
- Fat: 10g
- Carbohydrates: 58g
- Protein: 5g
- Cholesterol: 48mg

233. Cherry-Choco Bars

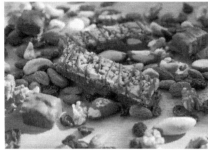

Preparation Time: 7 minutes
Cooking Time: 15 minutes
Servings: 8
Ingredients:
- ¼ tsp. salt
- ½ cup almonds, sliced
- ½ cup chia seeds
- ½ cup dark chocolate, chopped
- ½ cup dried cherries, chopped
- ½ cup prunes, pureed
- ½ cup quinoa, cooked
- ¾ cup almond butter
- 1/3 cup honey
- 2 cups oats
- 2 tbsp. coconut oil

Directions:
1. Preheat the fryer oven to 375°F.
2. Mix oats, quinoa, chia, almond, cherries, and chocolate.
3. Heat butter, honey, and oil in a saucepan.
4. Pour over the dry ingredients, add salt and prunes and mix completely.
5. Pour over an air-fitting baking dish.
6. Oven for 15 minutes
7. Cool before splitting into bars.

Nutrition:
- Calories: 100
- Fat: 4g
- Protein: 1g
- Cholesterol: 15mg

234. Crusty Apple Hand Pies

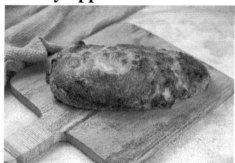

Preparation Time: 7 minutes
Cooking Time: 8 minutes
Servings: 6
Ingredients:
- 15-oz. no-sugar-added apple pie filling
- 1 store-bought crust

Directions:
1. Lay out the pie crust and slice it into equal-sized squares.
2. Place 2 tbsp. filling into each square and seal crust with a fork
3. Pour into the Oven rack/basket.
4. Place the rack on the middle shelf of the Smart Air Fryer Oven.
5. Set temperature to 390°F and set time to 8 minutes until golden in color.

Nutrition:
- 728 calories
- Protein 8.5g
- Carbohydrates 82.1g
- Fat 42g
- Cholesterol 61.8mg
- Sodium 753.9mg

235. Nutella-Stuffed Pancakes

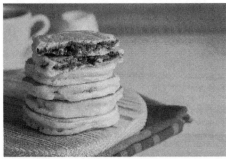

Preparation Time: 15 minutes
Cooking Time: 20 minutes
Servings: 12 pancakes
Ingredients:

- 1 tsp of chocolate-hazelnut spread, such as Nutella ®, at room temperature
- 1/4 cup vegetable oil, plus
- 1 1/4 cup grid all-purpose flour
- 1 1/4 cup buttermilk
- 1/4 cup of granulated Sugar
- 1 teaspoon baking soda
- 1 teaspoon baking soda
- 1 egg - A pinch of salt
- Sugar for dusting
- Maple syrup for serving

Directions:

1. Line a parchment baking sheet and drop 12 different teaspoonful mounds of chocolate hazelnut spread over it. Place the baking sheet on a counter to flatten the dollops and freeze for about 15 minutes until firm.
2. In the meantime, preheat a griddle over low heat and brush with oil lightly.
3. Whisk together flour, buttermilk, oil, granulated sugar, baking soda, egg, and a sprinkle of salt in a large bowl.
4. Pour batter pools on the hot griddle and cook until bubbles just start forming on the pancake's surface and the bottoms are golden, 1 to 2 minutes. Place a frozen chocolate hazelnut dish on 4 of the pancakes and turn over the remaining four pancakes so that the moist batter envelops the disks. Put the rest of the discs back into the freezer. Continue cooking the pancakes for about 1 minute, flipping halfway, until the edges are set. Repeat with the remaining batters and disks, oiling the grid lightly in between lots.
5. Stub the pancakes with the sugar of the confectioners and serve warmly with syrup.

Nutrition:

- Calories: 308
- Fat: 11g
- Carbohydrates: 46g
- Protein: 6g
- Cholesterol: 28mg

236. Chocolate Donuts

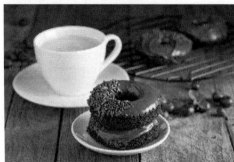

Preparation Time: 5 minutes
Cooking Time: 20 minutes
Servings: 8-10
Ingredients:

- (8-ounce) can jumbo biscuits
- Cooking oil
- Chocolate sauce, such as Hershey's

Directions:

1. Separate the dough into 8 biscuits and set it on a flat surface. Use a tiny circle cookie cutter to create a hole in the center of each biscuit. Use a knife to cut the holes.
2. Grease the basket with cooking oil.
3. Place 4 donuts in the Air Fryer oven. Do not stack. Spray with cooking oil. Cook for 4 minutes.
4. Open the fryer, turn the doughnuts. Cook another four minutes.
5. Remove the cooked donuts from the Air Fryer oven, then repeat for the remaining 4 donuts.
6. Drizzle chocolate sauce over the donuts and enjoy while warm.

Nutrition:

- Calories: 355
- Protein: 9 g
- Fat: 13 g
- Carbohydrates: 57 g

237. Blueberry Lemon Muffins

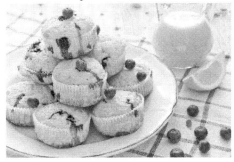

Preparation Time: 7 minutes
Cooking Time: 8 minutes
Servings: 12
Ingredients:
- 1 tsp. vanilla
- Juice and zest of 1 lemon
- 2 eggs
- 1 cup blueberries
- ½ cup cream
- ¼ cup avocado oil
- ½ cup monk fruit
- 2 ½ cups almond flour

Directions:
1. Mix fruit with flour.
2. Mix the meat and fruit.
3. In another bowl, mix vanilla, egg, citrus juice, and cream.
4. Stir completely with ingredients.
5. Bake for 8 minutes at 320°F on the Smart Air Fryer Oven check for 6 minutes to make sure it is not overbaked.

Nutrition:
- Calories: 265 Protein: 4.6g
- Carbohydrates: 39.7g Fat: 10.1g
- Cholesterol: 46.4mg
- Sodium: 339mg

238. Sweet Cream Cheese Wontons

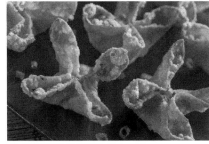

Preparation Time: 5 minutes
Cooking Time: 5 minutes
Servings: 16
Ingredients:
- 1 egg with a little water
- Wonton wrappers
- ½ cup powdered erythritol
- 8 oz softened cream cheese
- Olive oil

Directions:
1. Mix sweetener and cream cheese together.
2. Layout 4 wontons at a time and cover with a dish towel to prevent drying out.
3. Place ½ of a teaspoon of cream cheese mixture into each wrapper.
4. Dip finger into egg/water mixture and fold diagonally to form a triangle. Seal edges well.
5. Repeat with remaining ingredients.
6. Place filled wontons into the Air Fryer oven and cook 5 minutes at 400°F, shaking halfway through cooking.

Nutrition:
- Calories: 55
- Protein: 1 g
- Fat: 3 g
- Carbohydrates: 5 g
- Cholesterol: 11 mg

239. Saucy Fried Bananas

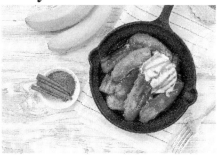

Preparation Time: 7 minutes
Cooking Time: 10 minutes
Servings: 2
Ingredients:
- 1 large egg
- ¼ cup cornstarch
- ¼ cup plain breadcrumbs
- Bananas halved crosswise
- Cooking oil
- Chocolate sauce

Directions:
1. Preheat the fryer oven to 350°F for your smart air.
2. Beat the egg in a bowl.
3. Put the starch in another bowl.
4. Place breadcrumbs in another bowl.
5. Pulp bananas, eggs, and breadcrumbs. Banana sprinkling.

6. Cooking oil spray basketball. Place bananas and oil spritz in the basket.
7. Five-minute cooking time.
8. Open the fryer, cook the bananas for another 2 minutes.
9. Take banana plates.
10. Serve the chocolate-sauce bananas.

Nutrition:
- Calories: 259
- Fat: 8g
- Carbohydrates: 46g
- Protein: 4g
- Cholesterol: 0 mg

240. Air-Fried Apple Pies

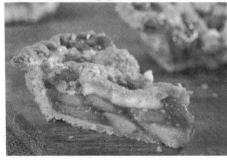

Preparation Time: 15 minutes
Cooking Time: 30 minutes
Servings: 4
Ingredients:
- 4 tbsp butter
- 6 tbsp brown sugar
- 1 tsp ground cinnamon
- 2 mediun Granny Smith apples, dices
- 1 tsp cornstarch
- 2 tsp cold-water
- Pastry (half of 1 - 14 oz. pkg. - for a 9-inch double-crust pie)
- Cooking spray
- ½ tbsp grapeseed oil
- ¼ cup powdered sugar
- Milk (1 tsp. + as needed)
- Suggested to use: A cast-iron skillet

Directions:
1. Dice and add the apples with the butter, brown sugar, and cinnamon in the skillet. Simmer them using the medium-temperature setting until apples have softened, about five minutes.
2. Dissolve cornstarch in cold water. Mix it into the apple mixture and simmer till the sauce thickens (1 min.). Transfer the pie filling from the burner and place it to the side to cool.
3. Unroll the pie on a floured surface.
4. Slice the dough into rectangles so that two can fit in the fryer basket at the same time.
5. Continue using the rest of the crust until you have eight equal rectangles, rerolling some of the dough scraps as needed.
6. Dampen the outer edges of four rectangles using a tiny bit of water and place some apple filling in the center about ½-inch from the edges.
7. Roll out the remaining four rectangles so that they are slightly larger than the filled ones.
8. Arrange them overfilling and close borders. Cut four small slits in the tops of the pies.
9. Spray the basket in the fryer unit with a cooking oil spray.
10. Lightly brush the tops of two pies with grape seed oil and transfer pies to the Air Fryer basket using a spatula.
11. Set the temperature to preheat at 385°F.
12. Bake until golden brown (8 min.). Transfer the pies from the basket and continue the process.
13. Mix the powdered sugar with the milk in a mixing container. Brush the glaze over the warm pies. Wait for the glazing to be slightly set.
14. Enjoy the pies while they're warm, or let them cool to enjoy later.

Nutrition:
- Calories: 497
- Protein: 3.2g
- Carbohydrates: 59.7g
- Fat: 28.6g
- Cholesterol: 30.5mg
- Sodium: 327.6mg

241. Air Fryer Tostones

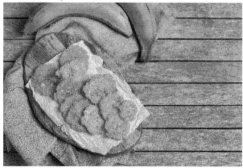

Preparation Time: 10 minutes
Cooking Time: 20 minutes
Servings: 4
Ingredients:
- 2 green unripe plantains

- 3 cups water, as needed
- Salt (as desired)
- Olive oil cooking spray

Directions:
1. Preheat the Air Fryer unit to reach 400° Fahrenheit/204° Celsius.
2. Remove the tips off the plantain. Make a vertical cut in the skin (end to end), not slicing into the plantain flesh.
3. With the peel attached, slice it into one-inch chunks. Peel the skin off each piece, starting at the slit you made.
4. Arrange the pieces in the basket and lightly spritz them with a tiny bit of cooking oil spray—Air-fry for five minutes.
5. Meanwhile, prepare a container of salted water.
6. Transfer the plantain pieces out of the fryer unit with tongs. Smash it to about a ½-inch thickness using a Costanera (plantain masher) to make the job more manageable if you have one. (It is an inexpensive tool found on Amazon.) If not, smash them with a fork.
7. Soak them in the salted water while mashing the rest.
8. Remove the water, patting them dry using a few paper towels.
9. Return the two stones to the Air Fryer in batches (single-layered).
10. Lightly spray the tops with a spritz of cooking oil spray and a dusting of salt. Air-fry them for five minutes.
11. Turn them over using tongs. Spritz the second side with additional oil spray.
12. Air-fry until golden brown and crispy to your liking (4-5 min.).

Nutrition:
- Carbohydrates: 28.5 g
- Fat: 04 g
- Protein: 1.2 g
- Calories: 109.8
- Sugar: 13.4 g
- Dietary Fiber: 2.1 g

242. Avocado-Chocolate Muffins

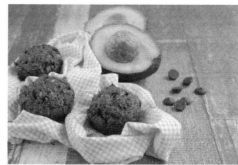

Preparation Time: 10 minutes
Cooking Time: 20 minutes
Servings: 7
Ingredients:
- 1 cup almond flour
- ½ tsp baking soda
- 1 tsp apple cider vinegar
- 1 egg
- 4 tbsp margarine
- 3 scoops Stevia powder
- ½ cup pitted avocado
- 1 oz melted dark chocolate

Directions:
1. Heat the Air Fryer to 355° Fahrenheit/179° Celsius.
2. Whisk the almond flour, baking soda, and vinegar.
3. Mix in the sweetener powder and melted chocolate.
4. Whisk the egg in another container and add to the mixture along with the butter.
5. Peel, cube, and mash in the avocado. Blend it all using a hand mixer to make the flour mixture is incorporated and smooth.
6. Pour into the muffin forms (½ full)—Cook for nine minutes.
7. Lower the heat (340° Fahrenheit/171° Celsius) and cook for three additional minutes.
8. Chill before serving for the most flavorful results.

Nutrition:
- Carbohydrates: 2.9 g
- Fat: 12.4 g
- Protein: 2.2 g
- Calories: 133

243. Banana Bread

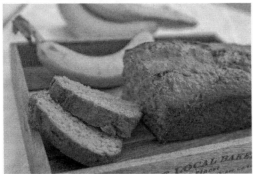

Preparation Time: 15 minutes
Cooking Time: 20 minutes
Servings: 8
Ingredients:

- ¾ cup / 3 oz white-whole wheat flour
- 1 tsp cinnamon
- ½ tsp Kosher salt
- ¼ tsp baking soda
- ¾ cup/2 medium/12 oz ripe bananas, mashed
- 2 large eggs
- ½ cup granulated sugar
- 1 tsp vanilla extract
- 1/3 plain nonfat yogurt
- 2 tbsp vegetable oil
- 2 tbsp./1/3 oz toasted walnuts, chopped
- Cooking spray
- Suggested: 5.3-quart Air Fryer
- Also needed: Six-inch round cake pan

Directions:

1. Cover the pan with parchment baking paper. Lightly coat the pan using a tiny bit of cooking oil spray.
2. Whisk the flour with the salt, cinnamon, and baking soda in a mixing container and set it aside for now. In a separate mixing container, beat the mashed bananas with the whisked eggs, sugar, yogurt, oil, and vanilla.
3. Gently combine the wet and dry ingredients until thoroughly combined. Empty the batter into the cake pan and sprinkle with walnuts.
4. Heat the fryer unit to 310° Fahrenheit/154° Celsius.
5. Arrange the pan in the fryer and air-fry until nicely browned and a wooden pick inserted in the middle comes out clean (30-35 min.), turning the pan halfway through cook time.
6. Move the bread to a wire rack to cool in the pan for 15 minutes before removing them from the pan and slicing.

Nutrition:

- Carbohydrates: 29 g Protein: 4 g
- Calories: 180 Sugar: 13 g
- Fiber: 2 g

244. Butter Cake

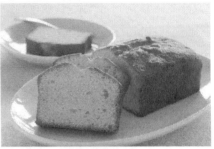

Preparation Time: 10 minutes
Cooking Time: 20 minutes
Servings: 1-4
Ingredients:

- Cooking spray, as neede
- 7 tbsp. unchilled butter
- ¼ cup + 2 tbsp. white sugar
- 1 egg
- 1 2/3 cups P. flour
- 1-2 pinches salt, to taste
- 6 tbsp. milk

Directions:

1. Preheat the Air Fryer to 350° Fahrenheit/177° Celsius.
2. Spray a small fluted tube pan with a spritz of cooking oil spray.
3. Combine the butter with all of the sugar using an electric mixer until it's creamy and light.
4. Whisk in the egg until incorporated. Fold in the salt and flour. Mix in the milk to form the batter.
5. Scoop the batter into the cake pan, using the back of a spoon to level the surface.
6. Put the pan in the fryer's basket. Set the timer for 15 minutes and bake until a toothpick inserted into the cake comes out clean.
7. Turn the cake off the pan and wait to cool (5 min.).

Nutrition:

- Carbohydrates: 59.7 g Fat: 22.4 g
- Protein: 7.9 g Calories: 470.2
- Sugar: 20.1 g Fiber: 1.4 g

245. Green Avocado Pudding

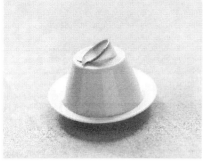

Preparation Time: 10 minutes
Cooking Time: 8-10 minutes
Servings: 3
Ingredients:

- 1 avocado, pitted
- 5 tbsp. almond milk - unsweetened
- 3 tsp. granulated sugar
- ¼ tsp. vanilla extract
- ¼ tsp. salt
- 1 tbsp. cocoa powder

Directions:

1. Heat the Air Fryer for a couple of minutes at 360° Fahrenheit/182° Celsius.
2. Peel and mash the avocado - combine with the milk, salt, vanilla extract, and sweetener. Stir in the cocoa powder.
3. Prepare in the Air Fryer for three minutes.
4. Chill well and serve.

Nutrition:

- Carbohydrates: 2.6 g
- Fat: 19.3 g
- Protein: 2.2 g
- Calories: 199

246. Cheesecake with Ricotta

Preparation Time: 15 minutes
Cooking Time: 25 minutes
Servings: 8
Ingredients:

- 17.6 oz. Ricotta cheese
- 3 eggs
- ¾ cup sugar
- 3 tablespoons corn starch
- 1 tablespoon fresh lemon juice
- 2 teaspoons vanilla extract
- 1 teaspoon fresh lemon zest, finely grated

Directions:

1. Preheat the Air Fryer to 320°F.
2. In a large bowl, place ricotta cheese, eggs, sugar, cornstarch, vanilla, lemon zest and juice, and mix until well combined.
3. Place mixture in a pan suitable for the Air Fryer.
4. Place the pan in the basket of the Air Fryer and bake for 25 minutes at 320°F.
5. Place the cake pan onto a wire rack to cool completely.
6. Refrigerate overnight before serving.

Nutrition:

- Calories: 97
- Fat: 6.6 g
- Carbohydrates: 15.7 g
- Protein: 92.2 g

247. Berry Crumble with Lemon

Preparation Time: 30 minutes
Cooking Time: 20 minutes
Servings: 6
Ingredients:

- 12 oz fresh strawberries
- 7 oz fresh raspberries
- 5 oz fresh blueberries
- 5 tbsp cold margarine
- 2 tbsp lemon juice
- 1 cup flour
- 1/2 cup sugar
- 1 tbsp water
- A pinch of salt (very little)

Directions:

1. Gently massage and chop berries, but make sure chunks remain.
2. Mix the berries with lemon juice and 2 tablespoons of sugar.
3. Place berry mixture in the bottom of a prepared round cake.
4. In a bowl, mix the flour with salt and sugar.
5. Add the water and rub in the margarine with your fingers until the mixture becomes crumbly.
6. Roll out the resulting dough and form it into a disk the width of your cake Pan or base.
7. Lay the crispy dough disk on top of the berries.
8. Bake in the deep fryer at 390°F for 20 minutes.

Nutrition:

- Calories: 250 Protein: 89.2 g
- Fat: 10.28 g
- Carbohydrates: 38.09 g

248. Apple Treat with Raisins

Preparation Time: 15 minutes
Cooking Time: 10 minutes
Servings: 4
Ingredients:

- 4 apples, cored
- 1 1/2 oz almonds
- ¾ oz raisins
- 2 tbsp sugar
- Powdered sugar, to taste

Directions:

1. Preheat Air Fryer to 360°F
2. In a bowl, mix sugar, almonds, raisins well.
3. Blend the mixture with a hand mixer.
4. Fill cored apples with almond mixture.
5. Place the prepared apples in the basket of the Air Fryer and bake for 10 minutes at 360°F. Serve with powdered sugar.

Nutrition:

- Calories: 188
- Protein: 72.88 g
- Fat: 5.64 g
- Carbohydrates: 35.63 g

249. French Toast Bites

Preparation Time: 5 minutes
Cooking Time: 15 minutes
Servings: 8
Ingredients:

- 1 cup almond milk
- 1 tbsp. cinnamon
- 2 tbsp. sweetener
- 3 eggs
- 4 pieces wheat bread

Directions:

1. Preheat the fryer to 360°F.
2. In a bowl, beat the eggs and dilute with the almond milk.
3. In another bowl mix 1/3 cup sweetener with plenty of cinnamon.
4. Cut the bread in half, knead the pieces, and press together to form bread balls
5. Dip the bread balls in the egg and then roll in the cinnamon sugar, making sure to coat completely.
6. Place the coated bread balls in the Air Fryer and bake for 15 minutes at 360°F.

Nutrition:

- Calories: 189 Protein: 49 g
- Fat: 11 g Carbohydrates: 17 g

250. Cinnamon Sugar Roasted Chickpeas

Preparation Time: 5 minutes
Cooking Time: 10 minutes
Servings: 2
Ingredients:

- 1 tbsp. sweetener
- 1 tbsp. cinnamon
- 1 cup chickpeas

Directions:

1. Preheat the fryer to 390°.
2. Rinse and drain chickpeas.
3. In a bowl, place drained chickpeas along with cinnamon, sweetener and mix everything to season the chickpeas well, and then place in the Air Fryer.
4. Set the temperature to 390°F and set the time to 10 minutes.
5. Serve and enjoy

Nutrition:

- Calories: 111
- Protein: 46 g
- Fat: 19 g
- Carbohydrates: 18 g

251. Brownie Muffins

Preparation Time: 10 minutes
Cooking Time: 10 minutes
Servings: 12
Ingredients:

- 1 package Betty Crocker fudge brownie mix
- 1/4 cup walnuts, chopped
- 1 egg
- 1/3 cup vegetable oil
- 2 teaspoons water
- 12 muffin molds

Directions:

1. Preheat the Air Fryer to 300°F.
2. Grease 12 muffin molds. Set aside.
3. In a bowl, put together walnuts, egg, vegetable oil, Betty Crocker fudge brownie mix, water, mix everything well.
4. Put the mixture into prepared muffin molds.
5. Place the muffin molds in the basket of the Air Fryer and bake for 10 minutes at 300°F.
6. Place the muffin molds onto a wire rack to cool for about 10 minutes.

7. Carefully, invert the muffins onto the wire rack to completely cool before serving.

Nutrition:
- Calories: 168 Protein: 72 g
- Fat: 8.9 g
- Carbohydrates: 20.8 g

252. Pear Sauce

Preparation Time: 10 minutes
Cooking Time: 20 minutes
Servings: 6
Ingredients:
- 10 pears, sliced
- 1 cup apple juice
- 1 ½ tsp cinnamon
- 1/4 tsp nutmeg

Directions:
1. Preheat the Air Fryer to 300°F.
2. Put pears, apple juice, cinnamon, nutmeg in the Air Fryer basket and stir well.
3. Place the basket in the Air Fryer and cook at 300°F for 20 minutes.
4. When finished cooking, allow to cool, and then blend the pear mixture with an immersion blender until smooth.
5. Serve and enjoy.

Nutrition:
- Calories: 222
- Protein: 91.3 g
- Fat: 0.6 g
- Carbohydrates: 58.2 g

253. Sweet Peach Jam

Preparation Time: 10 minutes
Cooking Time: 20 minutes
Servings: 20
Ingredients:
- 1 1/2 lb. fresh peaches, pitted and chopped
- 1/2 tbsp vanilla
- 1/4 cup maple syrup

Directions:
1. Preheat the Air Fryer to 350°F.
2. Put peaches, vanilla, maple syrup in the Air Fryer basket and stir well.
3. Place the basket inside the Air Fryer and cook at 350°F for 10 minutes, take out with a spoon, check to turn the mixture, and mix it by squeezing with the spoon. Put back in and cook for another 10 minutes at 350°F or until the jam has thickened.
4. Pour it into the container and store it in the fridge.

Nutrition:
- Calories: 16
- Protein: 91.1 g
- Fat: 0 g
- Carbohydrates: 3.7 g

254. Warm Peach Compote

Preparation Time: 10 minutes
Cooking Time: 5 minutes
Servings: 4
Ingredients:
- 4 peaches, peeled and chopped
- 1 tbsp water
- 1/2 tbsp cornstarch
- 1 tsp vanilla

Directions:
1. Add the water, vanilla, and peaches to the basket of the Air Fryer.
2. Place the basket inside and cook at 350°F for 5 minutes.
3. Pull out of Air Fryer
4. In a small bowl, whisk together 1 tablespoon water and cornstarch and pour into the pot and mix well.
5. Serve and enjoy.

Nutrition:
- Calories: 66 Protein: 51.4 g
- Fat: 0.4 g
- Carbohydrates: 15 g

255. Pan-Fried Bananas

Preparation Time: 15 minutes
Cooking Time: 8/12 minutes
Servings: 8
Ingredients:
- 8 bananas
- 3 tbsp vegetable oil
- 3 tbsp cornflour
- 1 egg white
- ¾ cup breadcrumbs
- Paper towels

Directions:
1. Preheat the Air Fryer on the toast function to 350°F.
2. Combine the oil and breadcrumbs in a bowl.
3. In another bowl, coat bananas with cornmeal, brush with egg white and dip in breadcrumb mixture.

4. Place on an Air Fryer-friendly baking sheet lined with paper towels and bake for 8-12 minutes at 350°F.

Nutrition:
- Calories: 162 Protein: 91.93 g
- Fat: 5.6 g
- Carbohydrates: 29.09 g

256. Blueberry Pudding

Preparation Time: 35 minutes
Cooking Time: 25 minutes
Servings: 6
Ingredients:
- 2 cups flour
- 2 cups rolled oats
- 8 cups blueberries
- 1 stick margarine
- 1 cup walnuts
- 3 tbsp. Maple syrup
- 2 tbsp. Rosemary

Directions:
1. Preheat the Air Fryer to 350°F.
2. Place blueberries in a pan suitable for the Air Fryer and spread over the entire surface of the pan.
3. In a bowl mix the rolled oats with the walnuts, flour, margarine, rosemary and maple syrup, whisk well, place the mix on top of the blueberries.
4. Place everything in the Air Fryer and bake at 350°F for 25 minutes.
5. Allow to cool, slice.

Nutrition:
- Calories: 278 Protein: 84.16 g
- Fat: 27.75 g Carbohydrates: 46 g

257. Banana-Choco Brownies

Preparation Time: 15 minutes
Cooking Time: 30 minutes
Servings: 12
Ingredients:
- 2 cups almond flour
- 2 + 1/2 teaspoons baking powder
- 1/2 teaspoon baking soda
- 1/2 teaspoon salt
- 1 over-ripe banana
- 3 large eggs
- 1/2 teaspoon stevia powder
- 1/4 cup coconut oil
- 1 tablespoon vinegar
- 1/3 cup almond flour
- 1/3 cup cocoa powder

Directions:
1. Preheat the Air Fryer for 5 minutes at 350°F.
2. Combine all ingredients in a food processor and blend until well combined and the mixture is smooth.
3. Pour into a pan that fits the Air Fryer.
4. Place in the fryer basket and bake for 30 minutes at 350°F or until a toothpick inserted in the center comes out clean.
5. Serve and enjoy

Nutrition:
- Calories: 75 Carbohydrates: 2.1 g
- Protein: 61.7 g Fat: 6.6 g

258. Dark Chocolate Oatmeal Cookies

Preparation Time: 10 minutes
Cooking Time: 8 to 13 minutes
Servings: 6
Ingredients:
- 3 tablespoons unsalted butter
- 2 oz dark chocolate, chopped
- 1/2 cup packed brown sugar
- 2 egg whites
- 1 teaspoon pure vanilla extract
- 1 cup quick-cooking oatmeal
- 1/2 cup whole-wheat pastry flour
- 1/2 teaspoon baking soda
- 1/4 cup dried cranberries

Directions:
1. In a medium metal bowl, mix butter and dark chocolate. Cook in the Air Fryer for 1 to 3 minutes at 360°F, or until butter and chocolate melts. Stir until smooth.
2. In a bowl, whisk the melted butter and chocolate into the brown sugar, egg whites, and vanilla until smooth.
3. Pour and stir in the oatmeal, pastry flour, and baking soda.
4. Pour and stir in the cranberries.
5. Form from the dough obtained about 30 balls (1 inch).
6. Bake the dough balls, in groups of 8, in the basket of the Air Fryer for 7-10 minutes at 370°F, or until cooked through.
7. Gently remove the cookies from the fryer and cool on a wire rack. Repeat with remaining dough balls.

Nutrition:
- Calories: 55 Fat: 2 g
- Protein: 81 g Carbohydrates: 8 g

259. Pumpkin Pie Pudding

Preparation Time: 10 minutes
Cooking Time: 12 to 17 minutes
Servings: 4
Ingredients:

- 1 cup canned no-salt-added pumpkin purée
- 1/4 cup packed brown sugar
- 3 tablespoons all-purpose flour
- 1 tablespoon unsalted butter, melted
- 1 egg
- 2 tablespoons 1 percent milk
- 1 teaspoon pure vanilla extract
- 4 low-fat vanilla wafers, crumbled

Directions:

1. Preheat the Air Fryer to 350°F.
2. Spray a pan suitable for the Air Fryer with nonstick cooking spray and set aside.
3. In a medium bowl, beat the pumpkin, brown sugar, flour, butter, egg, milk, and vanilla until combined and blended.
4. Pour the pumpkin mixture into the prepared pan.
5. Place in Air Fryer and bake for 12-17 minutes at 350°F, or until pudding is set and registers 165°F on a thermometer.
6. Remove the pudding from the Air Fryer and cool on a wire rack.
7. To serve, scoop the pudding into bowls and top with vanilla wafer crumbs.

Nutrition:

- Calories: 154
- Fat: 5 g
- Protein: 93 g
- Carbohydrates: 26 g

260. Apple Dumplings

Preparation Time: 15 minutes
Cooking Time: 25 minutes
Servings: 4
Ingredients:

- 2 tbsp. melted coconut oil
- 2 puff pastry sheets
- 1 tbsp. brown sugar
- 2 tbsp. raisins
- 2 small apples of choice

Directions:

1. Preheat the fryer to 356°F.
2. Core, peel and chop the apples and mix them in a bowl with the raisins and sugar.
3. Place some of the apple mixture into sheets of puff pastry and brush the sides with melted coconut oil.
4. Place in the Air Fryer. Bake 25 minutes at 356°F, turning halfway through baking. It will be golden brown when done.

Nutrition:

- Calories: 267 Fat: 7 g
- Protein: 92 g Sugar: 5 g

261. Cinnamon Fried Bananas

Preparation Time: 5 minutes
Cooking Time: 10/12 minutes
Servings: 2-3
Ingredients:

- 1 cup panko breadcrumbs
- 3 tbsp. cinnamon
- 1/2 cup almond flour
- 3 egg whites
- 8 ripe bananas
- 3 tbsp. vegan coconut oil

Directions:

1. Preheat the Air Fryer to 280°F.
2. Heat the coconut oil at 280°F for 2 minutes.
3. Take out and add the breadcrumbs to the oil. Stir about 2-3 minutes until golden brown.
4. Pour into a bowl.
5. Peel and cut the bananas in half.
6. In a bowl pour the flour and cinnamon and mix it, in another bowl beat the eggs whites.
7. Roll half of each banana first in flour mixture, then in eggs and then in crumbs and Place in lightly oiled fryer basket.
8. Bake for 10 minutes at 280°F.
9. Take out and serve.

Nutrition:

- Calories: 219
- Fat: 10 g
- Protein: 93 g
- Sugar: 5 g

262. Peanut Butter Chocolate Chip Cookies

Preparation Time: 5 minutes
Cooking Time: 12 minutes
Servings: 5
Ingredients:

- 1/2 cup peanut butter
- 1/4 cup turn sugar
- 1 egg yolk
- ½ tsp vanilla concentrate

- 1/8 tsp ocean salt
- ¼ cup Lily's dim chocolate chips
- Paper Towels

Directions:
1. Preheat your Air Fryer to 235°F and prepare the Air Fryer basket with paper towels.
2. Combine all ingredients in a large bowl until smooth and blended.
3. Scoop the batter onto the prepared plate and use a fork to mash it, making the peanut butter pattern on top.
4. Bake in the Air Fryer for 12 minutes at 235°F.
5. Allow to cool before serving

Nutrition:
- Calories: 185 Total Fat: 16 g
- Total Carbohydrates: 14 g Protein: 56 g

263. Chocolate Keto Cheesecake
Preparation Time: 15 minutes
Cooking Time: 1 hour 15 minutes
Servings: 12
Ingredients:
- 1/2-pound cream cheddar
- 5 tbsp margarine
- 1 cup powdered erythritol
- 1/4 cup unsweetened cocoa powder
- 3 eggs
- 1 1/2 tsp vanilla concentrate
- 3/4 cup harsh cream

Directions:
1. Preheat your Air Fryer to 275°F and oil an 8" spring-loaded pie plate. Also, place a piece of paper towel at the bottom of the pan.
2. Place the cream of cheddar and margarine in a huge bowl and whisk until consolidated and blended.
3. Add the erythritol powder, cocoa powder and beat again until smooth.
4. Add the eggs, one at a time, allowing them to fully blend after each serving.
5. Add the harsh cream and vanilla concentrate and mix one last time, making sure the beater is smooth and all the ingredients are heavily mixed and the mixture is smooth.
6. Empty the mixture into the prepared cake pan and then place it on a larger plate with high sides that will fit in the fryer.
7. Place in the preheated Air Fryer and cook for 1 hour and 15 minutes at 275°F.
8. Allow the cheesecake to cool for 3 hours in the cooler before removing it from the container and serving.

Nutrition:
- Calories: 302 Total Fat: 34 g
- Total Carbohydrates: 4 g Protein: 75 g

264. Vanilla Ciabatta Bread Pudding
Preparation Time: 15 minutes
Cooking Time: 20 minutes
Servings: 5
Ingredients:
- 1/2 cups ciabatta bread, cubed
- 2 eggs, whisked
- 1/2 cup double cream
- 1/2 cup milk
- 1/2 teaspoon vanilla extract
- 1/4 cup honey
- 1/2 cup golden raisins
- Spray oil

Directions:
1. Place the ciabatta bread in a lightly greased baking pan.
2. In a bowl, combine and thoroughly mix the eggs, heavy cream, milk, vanilla, and honey.
3. Pour the egg and cream mixture over the bread cubes. Add the raisins and set it aside for 15 minutes to soften.
4. Bake the bread pudding at 350°F for about 20 minutes or until the cream is set but still a little shaky.
5. Serve at room temperature. Serve and enjoy.

Nutrition:
- Calories: 217
- Fat: 7.3 g
- Carbohydrates: 34.6 g
- Protein: 65.1 g

265. Classic Baked Oatmeal
Preparation Time: 5 minutes
Cooking Time: 12 minutes
Servings: 4
Ingredients:
- 1 cup old-fashioned oats
- 1/4 cup agave syrup
- 1 cup milk
- 1 egg, whisked
- 1 cup apple, chopped
- 1/2 teaspoon baking powder
- 1/2 teaspoon ground cinnamon

- A pinch of grated nutmeg
- A pinch of salt (very little)
- Spray oil

Directions:
1. Preheat the Air Fryer to 380°F.
2. Thoroughly combine all ingredients in a mixing bowl.
3. Pour mixture into four lightly greased ramekins.
4. Next, place ramekins in the cooking basket of the Air Fryer.
5. Bake for about 12 minutes at 380°F.
6. Serve and enjoy.

Nutrition:
- Calories: 277
- Fat: 5.8 g
- Carbohydrates: 44.8 g
- Protein: 49.9 g

CHAPTER 14:

Liquid and Pureed Recipes

266. Alcohol-Free Mint Mojito

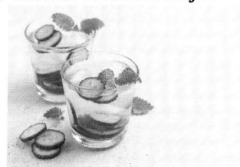

Preparation Time: 5 minutes
Cooking Time: 30 minutes
Servings: 4
Ingredients:
- 12/2 cup fresh mint leaves
- 1-ounce lime juice
- ½ cup natural sweetener
- 2 cups of water

Directions:
1. Add water and sweetener to a pot and let it boil for 5 minutes until the syrup has thickened.
2. Transfer mint leaves to a glass jar and pour them into the syrup.
3. Cover the jar and let it steep for 20 minutes.
4. Create a mixture of a tablespoon of the syrup and half a cup of cold water in a glass, add lime juice, and mix, serve and enjoy!

Nutrition:
- Calories: 32
- Total Fat: 0g
- Saturated Fat: 0g
- Protein: 0g
- Carbohydrates: 3g
- Fiber: 1g

267. Sugar-Free Strawberry Limeade

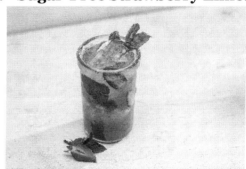

Preparation Time: 5 minutes
Cooking Time: 30 minutes
Servings: 4
Ingredients:
- ½ teaspoon strawberry extract
- 1 and ½ cups cold water
- Juice of ½ a lime

Directions:
1. Mix in strawberry extract, lime juice, and water in a bowl.
2. Take a cup and add ice cubes, pour the strawberry mixture and enjoy!

Nutrition:
- Calories: 12
- Total Fat: 0g
- Saturated Fat: 0g
- Protein: 1g
- Carbohydrates: 2.1g
- Fiber: 0.5g

268. Hearty Mint Tea

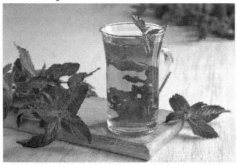

Preparation Time: 5 minutes
Cooking Time: 30 minutes
Servings: 4
Ingredients:

- 1-gallon boiling water
- 2 tablespoons mint
- 1 lemon, sliced
- 6 Rooibos tea bags

Directions:

1. Place water over high heat and let it start boiling.
2. Remove heat and add tea bags.
3. Pour the mixture into a pitcher (alongside tea bags, mint, and sliced lemon) and let it steep for 30 minutes.
4. Serve and enjoy!

Nutrition:

- Calories: 4
- Total Fat: 0g
- Saturated Fat: 0g
- Protein: 0.1g
- Carbohydrates: 1.4g
- Fiber: 0.1g

269. Orange and Apricot Juice

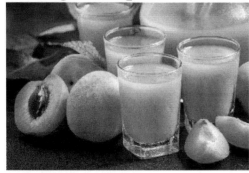

Preparation Time: 10 minutes
Cooking Time: 0 minutes
Servings: 2
Ingredients:

- 2 large oranges, peeled
- 2 large apricots, pitted
- 1 cup pomegranate seeds
- 1 cup of green grapes
- 1 large lemon, peeled
- 1 small ginger slice, peeled

Directions:

1. Peel oranges and divide them into wedges.
2. Keep them on the side.
3. Wash apricots and cut them in half, remove pits, and cut them into small pieces.
4. Cut the top of pomegranate fruit using a sharp knife and slice down each of the white membranes inside the fruit.
5. Pop seeds into a measuring cup and keep them on the side.
6. Peel the lemon and cut it lengthwise in half and keep it on the side.
7. Peel ginger slices and keep them on the side.
8. Add orange, apricots, pomegranate, lemon ginger to a juicer and process until well juiced.
9. Chill for 20 minutes and enjoy!

Nutrition:

- Calories: 196
- Total Fat: 0.8g
- Saturated Fat: 0g
- Protein: 4g
- Carbohydrates: 48g
- Fiber: 6.9g

270. Apple and Citrus Juice

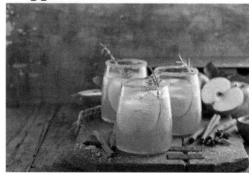

Preparation Time: 10 minutes
Cooking Time: 0 minutes
Servings: 2
Ingredients:

- 1 cup avocado, pitted and chopped
- 1 large cucumber, sliced
- 1 large lemon, peeled
- 1 cup fresh spinach, torn
- 1 large lime, peeled
- 1 small ginger knob, peeled
- 3 oz of water

Directions:
1. Peel your avocado and cut it in half. Remove pit and chop the avocado into chunks.
2. Wash the cucumber and cut it into thick slices.
3. Keep it aside.
4. Peel lemon and lime, cut their length in half.
5. Wash your spinach thoroughly and tear it into small parts.
6. Take your juicer and add avocado, cucumber, lemon, lime, spinach, ginger, and process until finely juiced.
7. Let it chill for 20 minutes, serve and enjoy!

Nutrition:
- Calories: 197
- Total Fat: 14g
- Saturated Fat: 3g
- Protein: 3g
- Carbohydrates: 19g
- Fiber: 8g

271. Blueberry Cacao Blast

Preparation Time: 2 minutes
Cooking Time: 3 minutes
Servings: 1
Ingredients:
- 1 cup blueberries
- 1 tbsp. raw cacao nibs
- 1 tbsp. chia seeds
- 1 dash cinnamon
- ½ cup chopped spinach
- ½ cup chopped bananas
- 1½ cup almond milk
- 2 scoops whey protein powder

Directions:
1. Place raspberries, cacao nibs, chia seeds, and cinnamon in a blender.
2. Add enough almond milk to reach the max line.
3. Process for 30 seconds or until you get a smooth mixture.
4. Serve immediately in a tall chilled glass.

Nutrition:
- Calories: 321 Carbohydrates: 69.4g
- Fat: 2.7g
- Protein: 24.7g

272. Cucumber and Avocado Dill Smoothie

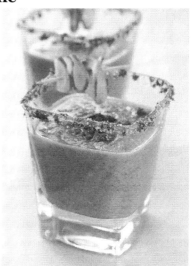

Preparation Time: 2 minutes
Cooking Time: 3 minutes
Servings: 2
Ingredients:
- 1 sliced cucumber
- 2 tbsps. chopped dill
- 2 tbsps. lemon juice
- 1 pitted avocado
- 1 cup coconut milk
- 1 tsp. shredded coconut
- 2 sliced kiwi fruit

Directions:
1. Mix and blend all the above ingredients using a blender. Drain the extract and discard residue. Serve and enjoy.

Nutrition:
- Calories: 165 Fat: 5.5g
- Carbohydrates: 24.8g Protein: 2.3g

273. Spinach Green Smoothie

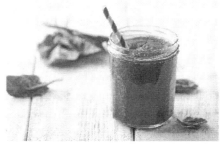

Preparation Time: 10 minutes
Cooking Time: 0 minutes
Servings: 2
Ingredients:
- 1 cup baby spinach leaves

- 3 mint leaves
- 1 cup 100% grapes juice
- 1 cup 100% pineapple juice
- 2 tbsps. lime juice
- 2 scoops protein powder

Directions:
1. In a blender, add the ingredients and blend well until puree.
2. Transfer to serving glasses.
3. Serve and enjoy.

Nutrition:
- Calories: 26 Fat: 5.5g
- Carbohydrates: 11.4g
- Protein: 24.3g

274. Coco - Banana Milkshake

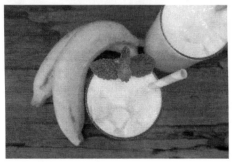

Preparation Time: 2 minutes
Cooking Time: 3 minutes
Servings: 1
Ingredients:
- 1 cup coconut milk
- 2 ripe bananas
- 2 tbsps. cinnamon
- ¼ tsp. cardamom powder
- 2 scoops protein powder
- 7 ice cubes

Directions:
1. In a blender add coconut milk with cardamom powder, cinnamon, bananas and blend well.
2. Pour into glass and add ice chunks. Serve and enjoy.

Nutrition:
- Calories: 191.9 Fat: 7.1g
- Carbohydrates: 35.8g
- Protein: 25.7g

275. Strawberry and Cherry Shake

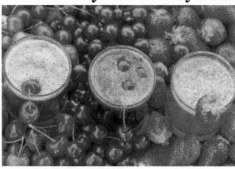

Preparation Time: 2 minutes
Cooking Time: 3 minutes
Servings: 2
Ingredients:
- 1 cup strawberries
- 1 cup cherries
- 1 cup almond milk
- ½ cup coconut milk
- 2 scoops protein powder
- A few blocks of ice

Directions:
1. Place all the ingredients in a blender and process well.
2. Serve and enjoy.

Nutrition:
- Calories: 138
- Fat: 0g
- Carbohydrates: 30g
- Protein: 20g

276. Chia Blueberry Banana Oatmeal Smoothie

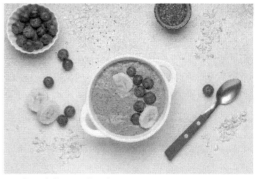

Preparation Time: 3 minutes
Cooking Time: 7 minutes
Servings: 1
Ingredients:
- 1 cup soy milk
- 1 sliced frozen banana
- ¼ cup frozen blueberries
- ¼ cup oats

- 1 tsp. vanilla extract
- 1 tsp. cinnamon
- 1 tbsp. chia seed

Directions:
1. Use a blender to mix and blend until the ingredients are combined and smooth.
2. Serve and enjoy!

Nutrition:
- Calories: 178
- Fat: 4.2g
- Carbohydrates: 36.2g
- Protein: 3.2g

277. Banana-Cherry Smoothie

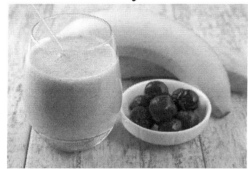

Preparation Time: 2 minutes
Cooking Time: 3 minutes
Servings: 1
Ingredients:
- 1 banana
- 1 cup pitted cherries
- ¼ tsp. nutmeg
- 1 scoop protein powder
- 1 cup almond milk

Directions:
1. Place all ingredients in a blender.
2. Process ingredients until smooth, for 20 seconds.
3. Serve immediately.

Nutrition:
- Calories: 398
- Fat: 2g
- Carbohydrates: 89.2g
- Protein: 17g

278. Mango Smoothie

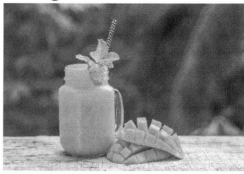

Preparation Time: 2 minutes
Cooking Time: 3 minutes
Servings: 2
Ingredients:
- 2 mangos (seeded, diced, frozen)
- 1 cup milk
- ½ cup crushed ice
- 1 cup plain yogurt
- 2 scoops protein powder

Directions:
1. Combine all ingredients in Vitamix.
2. Process for 30 seconds or until smooth.
3. Serve immediately in a tall glass.

Nutrition:
- Calories: 320
- Fat: 0g
- Carbohydrates: 8g
- Protein: 21g

279. Cashew Milk

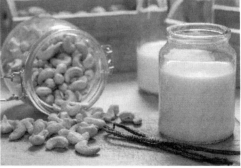

Preparation Time: 2 minutes
Cooking Time: 3 minutes
Servings: 5
Ingredients:
- 1 cup-soaked cashew
- 4 cup water
- 3 dates

Directions:
1. Add all ingredients to Vitamix.

2. Pulse until creamy (should take about 1 min).
3. Enjoy!

Nutrition:
- Calories: 60
- Fat: 2.5g
- Carbohydrates: 27.3g
- Protein: 8g

280. Pumpkin and Carrot Soup

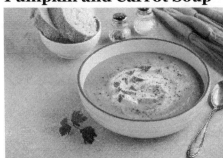

Preparation Time: 3 minutes
Cooking Time: 22 minutes
Servings: 4
Ingredients:
- ½ lb. pumpkin puree
- ½ lb. cubed carrots
- 2 cups vegetable stock
- ½ cup chopped onion
- Salt to taste
- Pepper to taste
- 1 tsp. dried thyme
- 2 oz. cauliflower florets
- ½ tbsp. olive oil
- 1 anise star

Directions:
1. Heat the oil in a pot. Add onion, cauliflower, carrots, and sauté for 15 minutes or until the onion is caramelized.
2. Add thyme and stir well.
3. Transfer the vegetables into a Nutri Bullet, add pumpkin puree and vegetable stock, and pulse until smooth.
4. Transfer the mixture into a saucepan and simmer, add anise star and simmer over medium-high heat for 5-8 minutes or until heated through.
5. Remove the anise star and discard.
6. Strain and serve immediately.

Nutrition:
- Calories: 70 Fat: 0g
- Carbohydrates: 0g
- Protein: 2g

281. Banana Almond Smoothie

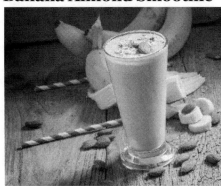

Preparation Time: 5 minutes
Cooking Time: 2 minutes
Servings: 1
Ingredients:
- 15 almonds
- 1 cup unsweetened almond milk
- 1 apple, peeled
- 1 banana, frozen

Directions:
1. Add all ingredients into the blender and blend until smooth and creamy.
2. Serve and enjoy.

Nutrition:
- Calories: 190 Fat: 5g
- Carbohydrates: 61g Sugars: 41g
- Protein: 14 g Cholesterol: 18 mg

282. Protein Spinach Shake

Preparation Time: 10 minutes
Cooking Time: 2 minutes
Servings: 1
Ingredients:
- 2/3 cup water
- ½ cup ice
- 5 drops liquid stevia
- ¼ cup vanilla protein powder
- ½ cup fat-free plain yogurt
- ½ tsp. vanilla extract
- 2 cups fresh spinach

Directions:
1. Add all ingredients into the blender and blend until smooth. Serve and enjoy.

Nutrition:
- Calories: 54 Fat: 0.9 g
- Carbohydrates: 14 g
- Fiber: 0 g Protein: 6 g
- Cholesterol: 0 mg

283. Fresh Lemon Cream Shake

Preparation Time: 5 minutes
Cooking Time: 2 minutes
Servings: 1
Ingredients:
- ½ cup ice cubes
- 2 tsp. lemon zest, grated
- ½ cup fat-free plain yogurt
- 1 scoop vanilla protein powder
- 5 oz. water
- 5 drops liquid stevia

Directions:
1. Add all ingredients into the blender and blend until smooth and creamy.
2. Serve and enjoy.

Nutrition:
- Calories: 175
- Fat: 0.1 g
- Carbohydrates: 9.8 g
- Fiber: 0 g
- Protein: 33.1 g
- Cholesterol: 4 mg

284. Avocado Banana Smoothie

Preparation Time: 10 minutes
Cooking Time: 2 minutes
Servings: 1
Ingredients:
- ½ tsp. vanilla
- 1 tbsp. honey
- 2 cups unsweetened coconut milk
- 1 cup ice cubes
- 1 cup baby spinach
- ½ avocado
- 3 bananas

Directions:
1. Add all ingredients into the blender and blend until smooth and creamy.
2. Serve and enjoy.

Nutrition:
- Calories: 425
- Fat: 33 g
- Carbohydrates: 33 g
- Fiber: 0 g
- Protein: 4 g
- Cholesterol: 0 mg

285. Banana Cherry Smoothie

Preparation Time: 5 minutes
Cooking Time: 2 minutes
Servings: 1
Ingredients:
- ½ tsp. vanilla
- 2 tbsp. unsweetened cocoa powder
- 2 ½ Tbsp. chia seeds
- 1 cup unsweetened almond milk
- 1 cup ice cubes
- 1 cup fresh spinach
- 1 banana

Directions:
1. Add all ingredients into the blender and blend until smooth and creamy.
2. Serve and enjoy.

Nutrition:
- Calories: 135
- Fat: 5 g
- Carbohydrates: 20 g
- Sugar: 7 g
- Protein: 4,6 g
- Cholesterol: 4 mg

286. Squash Soup

Preparation Time: 5 minutes
Cooking Time: 15 minutes
Servings: 1
Ingredients:
- 3 cups butternut squash, chopped
- 4 cups vegetable stock
- 3 garlic cloves, chopped
- 1 tbsp. olive oil
- 1 1/2 cups coconut milk
- 3/4 tbsp. curry powder
- 1/2 tsp. dried onion flakes
- 1 tsp. kosher salt

Directions:
1. Add butternut squash, oil, onion flakes, curry powder, stock, garlic, and salt into a saucepan and bring to a boil over medium-high heat.
2. Turn heat to medium and simmer for 20 minutes.
3. Puree the soup using an immersion blender until smooth.
4. Return soup to the saucepan and stir in coconut milk and cook for 2-3 minutes.

5. Serve and enjoy.

Nutrition:
- Calories: 144 Fat: 11g
- Carbohydrates: 10g Sugar: 2.5g
- Protein: 2 g Cholesterol: 0 mg

287. Creamy Avocado Soup

Preparation Time: 20 minutes
Cooking Time: 2 minutes
Servings: 1
Ingredients:
- 2 avocados, peel and pitted
- 2 cups vegetable stock
- 1 tbsp. fresh lemon juice
- 3/4 cup heavy cream
- 2 tbsp. dry sherry
- Pepper to taste
- Salt to taste

Directions:
1. Add avocado, lemon juice, sherry, and stock to the blender and blend until smooth.
2. Pour blended mixture into a bowl.
3. Add cream and stir well. Season with pepper and salt.
4. Serve and enjoy.

Nutrition:
- Calories: 102
- Fat: 9.5g
- Carbohydrates: 1.9g
- Sugar: 0.3g
- Protein: 2.4 g
- Cholesterol: 27 mg

288. Celery Soup

Preparation Time: 18 minutes
Cooking Time: 5 minutes
Servings: 1
Ingredients:
- 5 celery stalks, chopped
- 3 cups vegetable stock
- 3 tbsp. almonds, chopped
- Pepper to taste
- Salt to taste

Directions:
1. Add stock in a saucepan and bring to a boil over high heat for 2 minutes.
2. Add celery and cook for 8 minutes.
3. Remove from heat and use an immersion blender to puree until smooth.
4. Add almonds and stir well.
5. Season with pepper and salt.
6. Serve and enjoy.

Nutrition:
- Calories: 80
- Fat: 6g
- Carbohydrates: 5g
- Sugar: 2g
- Protein: 3 g
- Cholesterol: 0 mg

289. Cauliflower Soup

Preparation Time: 35 minutes
Cooking Time: 10 minutes
Servings: 1
Ingredients:
- ½ head cauliflower, chopped
- 2 garlic cloves, minced
- 15 oz. vegetable stock
- ¼ tsp. garlic powder
- 1 onion, diced
- 1 tbsp. olive oil
- ¼ tsp. pepper
- ½ tsp. salt

Directions:
1. Heat oil in a saucepan over medium heat.
2. Add onion and garlic and sauté for 4–5 minutes.
3. Add cauliflower and stock and stir well. Bring to a boil.
4. Cover and simmer for 15 minutes. Season with garlic powder, pepper, and salt.
5. Puree the soup using a blender until smooth.
6. Serve and enjoy.

Nutrition:
- Calories: 40
- Fat: 2g
- Carbohydrates: 4g
- Sugar: 2g
- Protein: 3 g
- Cholesterol: 0 mg

290. Avocado Milk Whip

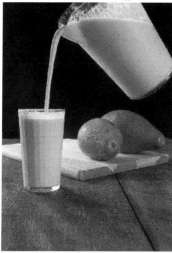

Preparation Time: 10 minutes
Cooking Time: 0 minutes
Servings: 1
Ingredients:
- 1 avocado, peeled, pitted, diced
- 1 cup skimmed milk
- ½ cup non-fat cottage cheese
- ¼ cup fresh cilantro leaves, stems removed
- ½ teaspoon lime juice
- ¼ teaspoon garlic powder
- Chili powder, for garnish

Directions:
1. Put all ingredients in a blender and blend until smooth.
2. Divide the whip between two bowls and sprinkle with a dash of chili powder to serve.

Nutrition:
- Calories: 317
- Fat: 20g
- Carbohydrates: 26.6g
- Sugar: 17.7g
- Protein: 2 g
- Cholesterol: 0 mg

291. Banana and Kale Smoothie

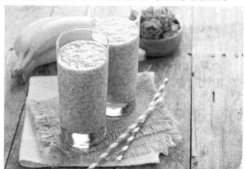

Preparation Time: 5 minutes
Cooking Time: 0 minutes
Servings: 1
Ingredients:
- 2 cups unsweetened almond milk
- 2 cups kale, stemmed, leaves chopped
- 2 bananas, peeled
- 1 to 2 packets stevia, or to taste
- 1 teaspoon ground cinnamon
- 1 cup crushed ice

Directions:
1. In a blender, combine the almond milk, kale, bananas, stevia, cinnamon, and ice. Blend until smooth.
2. Serve immediately.

Nutrition:
- Calories: 181
- Fat: 4g
- Carbohydrates: 37g
- Sugar: 15g
- Protein: 4 g
- Cholesterol: 0 mg

292. Beef Purée

Preparation Time: 30 minutes
Cooking Time: 2-5 hours
Servings: 1
Ingredients:
- 1 pound (454 g) beef tenderloin steak
- 1 teaspoon olive oil
- 1 teaspoon soy sauce
- ½ teaspoon salt, plus more to taste
- ½ teaspoon garlic powder
- ½ teaspoon onion powder
- ½ teaspoon dried rosemary, crushed
- ½ teaspoon dried parsley

- ¼ teaspoon freshly ground black pepper, plus more to taste
- Beef stock, as needed

Directions:
1. Pat the steak dries with paper towels and brush with olive oil and soy sauce. Mix salt, garlic powder, onion powder, rosemary, parsley, and pepper and rub over steak. Cook the steak in a slow cooker until cooked through and the internal temperature reaches 145°F (63°C), 8 to 10 hours at the low setting or 4 to 5 hours at the high setting.
2. Remove the steak from the slow cooker, reserving the cooking juices. Put the steak in a covered container and refrigerate until chilled through, about 2 hours.
3. Cut the chilled steak into 1-inch cubes. Put about 1 cup steak cubes in a food processor and blend until fine and powdery. Add about ¼ cup reserved cooking juices plus stock as needed and process until smooth. Repeat with remaining steak cubes. Season the puréed steak with salt and pepper and stir until thoroughly combined.
4. Serve immediately.

Nutrition:
- Calories: 168 Fat: 7.9g
- Carbohydrates: 1g Sugar: 0.3g
- Protein: 23.3 g Cholesterol: 0 mg

293. Blueberry and Spinach Smoothie

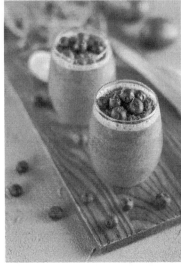

Preparation Time: 5 minutes
Cooking Time: 2 minutes
Servings: 1
Ingredients:
- 2 cups blueberries
- 3 cups chopped fresh spinach
- ½ cup chopped fresh coriander
- Juice of 1 lemon
- 1-inch fresh ginger, grated
- 2 cups water

Directions:
1. Put all the ingredients in the blender, mix for 2 minutes or until smooth.
2. Serve immediately.

Nutrition:
- Calories: 121
- Fat: 0.6g
- Carbohydrates: 30g
- Sugar: 26.6g
- Protein: 1.6 g
- Cholesterol: 0 mg

294. Broccoli Purée

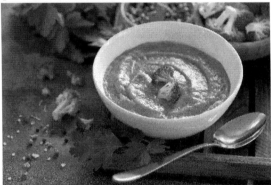

Preparation Time: 30 minutes
Cooking Time: 5 minutes
Servings: 1
Ingredients:
- 1 pound (454 g) fresh broccoli, cut into florets
- ½ cup water
- ½ teaspoon salt, plus more to taste
- 1 teaspoon butter
- 1 teaspoon lemon juice
- ½ teaspoon onion powder
- Freshly ground black pepper, to taste

Directions:
1. Mix the broccoli florets, water, and ½ teaspoon salt in a medium saucepan and bring to a simmer. Reduce heat, cover the pan and simmer until the broccoli is tender, 5 to 10 minutes.
2. Drain the broccoli, reserving the cooking water. Add the butter, lemon juice, and onion powder, season with salt and pepper, and let cool.

3. Put about 1 cup broccoli florets and ¼ cup cooking water in a food processor and mix until smooth. Repeat with remaining broccoli.
4. Serve immediately.

Nutrition:
- Calories: 28 Carbohydrates: 4.3g
- Protein: 2.4g Fat: 0.9g
- Sugar: 1.g Fiber: 2.3g
- Sodium: 212mg

295. Easy Chocolate and Orange Pudding

Preparation Time: 5 minutes
Cooking Time: 5 minutes
Servings: 1
Ingredients:
- 1 package sugar-free instant chocolate pudding mix
- ¼ cup chocolate protein powder
- 2 cups low-fat milk
- 1 tablespoon cocoa powder
- 1 teaspoon orange extract

Directions:
1. In a small bowl, whisk the pudding and protein powders together with the milk for 2 minutes.
2. Add the cocoa powder and orange extract, and mix for 3 more minutes before serving.

Nutrition:
- Calories: 11
- Carbohydrates: 15g
- Protein: 10g
- Fat: 2g Sugar: 6g
- Fiber: 1g
- Sodium: 380mg

296. Herbed Chicken Purée

Preparation Time: 30 minutes
Cooking Time: 15 minutes
Servings: 1
Ingredients:
- 2 (8-ounce / 227-g) boneless skinless chicken breasts
- 2 bay leaves
- ¾ teaspoon salt, divided
- ¾ teaspoon ground sage
- ½ teaspoon ground thyme
- ¼ teaspoon ground marjoram
- ¼ teaspoon ground rosemary
- ¼ teaspoon freshly ground black pepper
- Dash of nutmeg

Directions:
1. Put the chicken breasts, bay leaves, and 1/2 teaspoon in a medium saucepan, add enough cold water to cover, and bring to a boil. Reduce the heat, cover, and simmer gently until chicken is cooked through and the internal temperature reaches at least 165°F (74°C), 20 to 25 minutes.
2. Remove the chicken breasts from the broth. Strain and reserve the broth. Put chicken in a covered container and refrigerate until chilled through, about 2 hours.
3. Cut the chilled chicken breasts into 1-inch cubes. Put about 1 cup chicken cubes in a food processor and pulse until fine and powdery. Add about ¼ cup reserved broth and process until smooth. Repeat with remaining chicken cubes.
4. Mix the sage, thyme, marjoram, rosemary, pepper, and nutmeg with remaining salt, sprinkle over the puréed chicken, and stir until thoroughly combined. Serve immediately.

Nutrition:
- Calories: 92 Carbohydrates: 0.2g
- Protein: 17.1g Fat: 2g
- Sugar: 0g Fiber: 0.1g Sodium: 325mg

297. Matcha Mango Smoothie

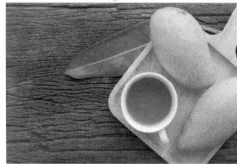

Preparation Time: 5 minutes
Cooking Time: 0 minutes
Servings: 1
Ingredients:
- 2 cups cubed mango
- 2 tablespoons matcha powder
- 2 teaspoons turmeric powder
- 2 cups almond milk
- 2 tablespoons honey
- 1 cup crushed ice

Directions:
1. In a blender, combine the mango, matcha, turmeric, almond milk, honey, and ice. Blend until smooth.

2. Serve immediately.

Nutrition:
- Calories: 285 Carbohydrates: 68 g
- Protein: 4 g Fat: 3 g Sugar: 63 g Fiber: 6 g
- Sodium: 94 mg

298. Ricotta Peach Fluff

Preparation Time: 10 minutes
Cooking Time: 0 minutes
Servings: 1
Ingredients:
- ¼ cup ricotta cheese
- 1 ripe peach, diced
- 2 tbsp. skim milk

Directions:
1. Purée ricotta, diced peach, and milk in a blender until smooth. Serve immediately

Nutrition:
- Calories: 355
- Carbohydrates: 54 g Protein: 17.9 g
- Fat: 8.7 g Sugar: 50 g
- Fiber: 2 g
- Sodium: 183 mg

299. Split Pea and Carrot Soup

Preparation Time: 10 minutes
Cooking Time: 1 hour 10 minutes
Servings: 1
Ingredients:
- 1 tbsp. extra-virgin olive oil
- 2 large carrots, chopped
- 1 medium onion, diced
- 2 garlic cloves, minced
- 4 cups chicken broth
- 2 cups water
- Salt, to taste
- Freshly ground black pepper, to taste
- 2 dried bay leaves
- 1 (16-ounce / 454-g) bag green split peas

Directions:
1. In a large stockpot over medium heat, heat the oil.
2. Add the carrot, onion, and garlic. Sauté until soft, 5 to 7 minutes.
3. Add the broth, water, salt and pepper, bay leaves, and split peas. Stir well, and bring to a boil.
4. Reduce the heat to a simmer, cover, and let cook for 1 hour, or until the peas are soft.
5. Remove the bay leaves, and serve immediately.

Nutrition:
- Calories: 92
- Carbohydrates: 20 g
- Protein: 8 g
- Fat: 1 g
- Sugar: 2 g
- Fiber: 8 g
- Sodium: 264 mg

300. Herb And Melon Kefir Smoothie

Preparation Time: 10 minutes
Cooking Time: 15 minutes
Servings: 1
Ingredients:
- 4 oz nonfat plain kefir
- ¼ cup nonfat plain Greek yogurt
- ¾ cup chopped honeydew melon
- 4 fresh mint leaves
- 2 fresh basil leaves
- 1 teaspoon honey
- ¼ teaspoon vanilla extract

Directions:
1. In a blender, combine the kefir, yogurt, melon, mint, basil, honey, and vanilla.
2. Blend until smooth, or until your desired consistency is reached. Pour into a glass and enjoy.

Nutrition:
- Calories: 159
- Carbohydrates: 26 g
- Protein: 11 g
- Fat: 2 g
- Sugar: 25 g
- Fiber: 6 g
- Sodium: 94 mg

301. Kefir And Yogurt Banana Flaxseed Shake

Preparation Time: 10 minutes
Cooking Time: 8 minutes to chill
Servings: 1
Ingredients:
- 1/3 cup nonfat plain kefir
- 6 oz nonfat plain Greek yogurt
- ½ banana, fresh or frozen
- 1 tablespoon ground flaxseed

- 1 tablespoon sunflower seed butter
- 1 teaspoon sugar-free vanilla syrup or honey (optional)

Directions:
1. In a blender, combine the kefir, yogurt, banana, flaxseed, sunflower seed butter, and syrup (if using).
2. Blend until smooth. Pour into a glass and enjoy.
3. Alternatively, refrigerate for 10 to 15 minutes to chill before sipping.

Nutrition:
- Calories: 329
- Carbohydrates: 28 g
- Protein: 26 g
- Fat: 14 g
- Sugar: 17 g
- Fiber: 0 g
- Sodium: 157 mg

302. Piña Colada Smoothie

Preparation Time: 10 minutes
Cooking Time: 8 minutes to chill
Servings: 1
Ingredients:
- ½ cup canned pineapple chunks, drained
- 4 oz unsweetened coconut milk
- ½ cup nonfat plain Greek yogurt
- ½ teaspoon coconut extract

Directions:
1. In a blender, combine the pineapple, coconut milk, yogurt, and coconut extract.
2. Blend until smooth, or until your desired consistency is reached. Pour into a glass and enjoy.
3. Alternatively, refrigerate for 10 to 15 minutes to chill before sipping.

Nutrition:
- Calories: 148 Carbohydrates: 19 g
- Protein: 13 g Fat: 3 g
- Sugar: 17 g Fiber: 1 g
- Sodium: 46 mg

303. Green Mango Smoothie

Preparation Time: 10 minutes
Cooking Time: 2 minutes
Servings: 1
Ingredients:
- 1/3 avocado, peeled and pitted
- 1/3 cup fresh spinach
- ½ cup canned mango chunks, drained
- ½ cup nonfat plain Greek yogurt
- ½ cup nonfat milk
- 1 teaspoon honey or sugar-free vanilla syrup

Directions:
1. In a blender, combine the avocado, spinach, mango, yogurt, milk, and honey.
2. Blend until smooth, or until your desired consistency is reached. Pour into a glass and enjoy.

Nutrition:
- Calories: 261 Carbohydrates: 30 g
- Protein: 21 g Fat: 8 g
- Sugar: 63 g Fiber: 6 g Sodium: 117 mg

304. Peachy Greek Yogurt Panna Cotta

Preparation Time: 10 minutes
Cooking Time: 5 minutes & 2-8 hours to chill
Servings: 1
Ingredients:
- ½ cup nonfat milk
- 1½ tablespoon honey
- 1 tablespoon unflavored powdered gelatin
- 1½ cup nonfat plain Greek yogurt
- ½ teaspoon vanilla extract (optional)
- ½ cup canned no-sugar-added sliced peaches, drained

Directions:
1. In a small saucepan over low heat, heat the milk for 2 to 4 minutes until lukewarm. Add the honey and gelatin. Cook for 3 to 5 minutes, stirring, until the honey and gelatin dissolve. (Do not bring to a boil.) Remove from the heat.
2. In a small bowl, whisk the yogurt until smooth. Add the warm gelatin mixture and vanilla (if using). Whisk well to combine. Pour into 4 small jars, glasses, or ramekins. Refrigerate for at least 2 hours or overnight for best results.
3. Before serving, put the canned peaches into a blender or food processor and puree until smooth.
4. Top each panna cotta with 2 tablespoons of pureed peach and enjoy.

Nutrition:
- Calories: 106
- Carbohydrates: 13 g
- Protein: 12 g Fat: 1 g
- Sugar: 13 g
- Fiber: 1 g
- Sodium: 48 mg

305. Nutty Creamy Wheat Bowl

Preparation Time: 5 minutes
Cooking Time: 5 minutes
Servings: 1
Ingredients:

- 4 oz. nonfat milk
- 1 tablespoon uncooked Cream of Wheat
- Salt to taste
- 1 teaspoon almond butter
- Ground cinnamon, for seasoning
- ½ banana, mashed

Directions:

1. In a small saucepan or pot, stir together the milk and Cream of Wheat until combined. Place the pot over medium-high heat and bring the mixture to a boil, whisking frequently to keep lumps from forming.
2. Reduce the heat to low and simmer the cereal for 1 to 2 minutes, just until it thickens. Season with salt to taste and pour the cereal into a bowl.
3. Add the almond butter and season with cinnamon. Top the cereal with mashed banana before enjoying.

Nutrition:

- Calories: 167 Carbohydrates: 26 g
- Protein: 10 g Fat: 3 g
- Sugar: 11 g Fiber: 0 g
- Sodium: 127 mg

CHAPTER 15:

30 Days Meal Plan

Day	Breakfast	Lunch	Snack	Dinner
1	Tuna Sandwiches	Easy Rosemary Lamb Chops	Tacos Crispy Avocado	Brine-Soaked Turkey
2	Garlic Potatoes with Bacon	Greek Lamb Chops	Apple chips with cinnamon and yogurt sauce	Spicy Catfish
3	Chicken & Zucchini Omelet	Easy Beef Roast	Mozzarella Cheese Bites with Marinara Sauce	Thyme Turkey Breast
4	Tomatoes and Swiss Chard Bake	Juicy Pork Chops	Spanakopita Bites	Chicken Drumsticks
5	Shrimp Frittata	Tuna and Spring Onions Salad	Kale Chips – Vegan-Friendly	Mushroom Pita Pizzas
6	Zucchini Fritters	Bacon-Wrapped Filet Mignon	Light air-fried Empanadas	Parmesan Chicken Meatballs
7	Chicken Omelet	Classic Beef Jerky	Whole-Wheat Air-Fried Pizzas	Easy Italian Meatballs
8	Scrambled Eggs	Flavorful Steak	Zucchini Chips	Buttered Salmon
9	Almond Crust Chicken	BBQ Pork Chops	Air-Fried Avocado Fries	Simple Haddock
10	Mushroom Cheese Salad	Crispy Meatballs	Chicken Nachos with Pepper	Miso Glazed Salmon
11	Shrimp Sandwiches	Juicy Steak Bites	Dark Chocolate and Cranberry Granola Bars	Split Pea and Carrot Soup
12	Mushrooms and Cheese Spread	Lemon Garlic Lamb Chops	Bacon Muffin Bites	Lemony Salmon
13	Lemony Raspberries Bowls	BBQ Pork Ribs	Brussels Sprout Chips	Creamy Potatoes
14	Asparagus Salad	Herb Butter Rib-eye Steak	Herbed Parmesan Crackers	Vinegar Halibut
15	Zucchini Squash Mix	Honey Mustard Pork Tenderloin	Cauliflower Crunch	Crusted Chicken Drumsticks
16	Bacon-Wrapped Filet Mignon	Simple Beef Sirloin Roast	Lemon Pepper Broccoli Crunch	Spiced Tilapia
17	Pumpkin Pancakes	Seasoned Beef Roast	Delicate Garlic Parmesan Pretzels	Ricotta Peach Fluff
18	Onion Omelet	Beef Burgers	Cucumber Chips	Breaded Cod

19	Sweetened Breakfast Oats	Season and Salt-Cured Beef	Cajun Cauliflower Crunch	Eggs with Veg
20	Veggie Quiche Muffins	Simple Beef Patties	Sprouts Wraps	Tuna Burgers
21	Steel Cut Oat Blueberry Pancakes	Baked Tilapia Cheese	Pickled Bacon Bowls	Lentils with Mushrooms
22	Very Berry Muesli	Breaded Cod Sticks	Curried Brussels Sprouts	Turkey Meatballs
23	Strawberry & Mushroom Breakfast Sandwich	Shrimp, Zucchini and Cherry Tomato Sauce	Crispy Cauliflower Bites	English Muffin Tuna Sandwiches
24	Shakshuka Egg Bake	Honey Glazed Salmon	Garlic Asparagus	Pesto Gnocchi
25	Ricotta Baked in The Oven	Crumbled Fish	Crispy Kale Chips	Crispy Prawns
26	Poached Eggs Italian Style	Salted Marinated Salmon	Crispy Squash	Sweet & Spicy Meatballs
27	Denver Egg Muffins with Ham Crust	Sautéed Trout with Almonds	Garlic Mozzarella Sticks	Vegetable Egg Rolls
28	Cheesy Slow Cooker Egg Casserole	Cod Fish Nuggets	Homemade Peanut Corn Nuts	Steak With Cheese Butter
29	Tuna Sandwiches	Creamy Salmon	Divided Balsamic Mustard Greens	Potatoes with Black Beans
30	Garlic Potatoes with Bacon	Baked Onion Cod	Honey Roasted Carrots	Lentils with Mushrooms

Conclusion

The Bariatric Diet is a weight-loss surgery that includes a high-protein, low-calorie diet. It has been in place in European hospitals for more than 40 years. When the digestive system is unable to adequately process foods or when an individual needs to reduce weight quickly, there are many different types of diets available.

This type of diet is the only surgery available for people with life-threatening obesity who are also at risk for developing diabetes, heart disease, and other serious health problems. The bariatric diet has been around for a long time, but it is only recently that the diet was introduced to the medical community.

A lot of people have lost weight with the Bariatric Diet. For some people, this has meant a few pounds and for others, it is enough to save their lives.

There are two kinds of Bariatric Diets: one that is completely liquid, and another that includes solid foods. Both types of diets involve eating smaller portions that are low in calories and made up of mostly protein and very little fat.

The Bariatric Liquid Diet is designed for patients who have difficulty chewing and swallowing. It consists of foods that are easily liquefied, such as chicken broth, applesauce, and vanilla ice cream. It contains at least 1,200 calories and is crucial when the patient goes home after surgery. The Bariatric diet usually lasts between 18 to 24 months and it ends before the patient transitions to the Maintenance Diet which is the standard weight-loss diet plan.

The Bariatric solid food diet has at least 500 calories per meal. The meals are larger and are usually based on the main course, side dishes, and drinks. The solid food diet is good for people who want to lose weight but prefer not to go under the knife. Vitals and blood tests are done to ensure that nothing has changed during the time of the surgery.

The goal of bariatric surgery is weight loss. It takes years for the patient to achieve this goal, but it is safer than other treatments, like gastric bypass or gastric sleeve surgery because it does not require any major changes in lifestyle. In fact, after the procedure, almost all of these patients eat as if they had never undergone an operation at all.

The Bariatric Surgery Diet focuses on calories in versus calories out. With the Bariatric Diet, small, frequent meals are prescribed. If the patient is interested in getting on the Maintenance Diet, a Physician Assistant or physician will suggest a menu. The patients in this diet plan are motivated to eat healthy foods by enjoying all of their favorite foods and drinks as if they were weight-neutral.

All of the patient's dietary and liquid input is monitored every day. The Bariatric Diet is also known as a Pre-Op Diet and a Pre-Op Weight Loss Program.

Obesity disease can be prevented or treated with lifestyle changes, according to the medical community. This is known as making lifestyle changes. Lifestyle change means making many positive changes in diet and exercise habits.

Manufactured by Amazon.ca
Bolton, ON